{ How to Survive Your Bad Habits }

The Healthy Guide to Unhealthy Living

David J. Clayton, M.D.,
with Laura Vanderkam

Simon & Schuster Paperbacks

New York London Toronto Sydney

The information and suggestions contained in this book cannot substitute for proper medical care. Consult your doctor or other health care provider before adopting the suggestions in this book. The authors and publisher disclaim any liability arising directly or indirectly from the use of this book.

SIMON & SCHUSTER PAPERBACKS
Rockefeller Center
1230 Avenue of the Americas
New York, NY 10020

First Simon & Schuster paperback edition 2006

SIMON & SCHUSTER PAPERBACKS and colophon are registered
trademarks of Simon & Schuster, Inc.

For information about special discounts for bulk purchases,
please contact Simon & Schuster Special Sales:
1-800-456-6798 or business@simonandschuster.com.

Book design by Ellen R. Sasahara

Manufactured in the United States of America

2 4 6 8 10 9 7 5 3 1

Library of Congress Cataloging-in-Publication Data
Clayton, David J.
The healthy guide to unhealthy living : [how to survive your bad habits] / David J.
Clayton with Laura Vanderkam.
p. cm.
Includes index.
1. Health behavior–Popular works. 2. Self-care, Health–Popular works.
3. Health–Popular works. I. Vanderkam, Laura. II. Title.
RA776.9.C55 2006
613–dc22   2005049967

ISBN-13: 978-0-7432-7214-8
ISBN-10:   0-7432-7214-5

Contents

The Healthy Guide to Unhealthy Living

Introduction

DESPITE all the self-help books out there on living a healthy life, many of my patients don't want to know how to live a healthy life–they want to know how to live their unhealthy lives better.

They don't want to stop drinking, smoking, doing drugs, or having casual sex with the other sleep-deprived professionals they meet at parties. They want to know how to do these things without killing themselves or permanently damaging their health. They want to know how to lose weight fast for a wedding, or whether a drug test will show last week's joint. They want to know how to stay awake at the office when they haven't slept well the night before.

I began mulling over a manual on bad habits when I moved to New York after finishing my residency in internal medicine in San Diego. In the hospital where I worked on the West Coast, most of my patients were over seventy. I learned a lot by helping them manage such problems as congestive heart failure, stroke, kidney and lung disease, but I also spent a lot of heart-wrenching hours trying to console the families of dying patients.

New York was completely different. After my residency, I headed to the Big Apple to study business at Columbia. I needed cash to put myself through school, so I landed a job at a medical clinic on the Upper East Side.

At this clinic, my patients were closer to age thirty than eighty. Virtually no one had a chronic disease, and the few who did were intelligent and motivated enough to partner with me in treating their illnesses. Most of my clients were professional bankers, lawyers, or consultants, and I even had a celebrity come through now and then. After earning my MBA, I started my own practice and kept seeing high-octane young professionals along with those just moving to New York ready to make their mark on the town.

The one thing that rich bankers and struggling actors have in common in New York, I discovered, is their desire to make the most of their lives. New Yorkers always want more than they have. Everyone is trying to make it here. To make it, people will push themselves beyond a sane, sensible existence. You don't have to be a doctor to know that eighteen-hour days in the office and happy hours that last until dawn wear on the body.

I call these young people the "worried well." They suspect their habits are unhealthy, but they don't know what to do about them. I don't blame them for the confusion. Even with all the medical books out there, the Internet, and TV doctors galore, nonpreachy information on drugs or sexually transmitted diseases is hard to come by. The Internet just tells you that bump could be AIDS, or that burning could be chlamydia, herpes, gonorrhea, or ten other diseases, and next thing you know, you're a quivering mess. TV doctors tell you to stop screwing around and see your own doctor. When you get that appointment four itchy days later, he'll say that you may have caught something, but the cultures won't come back from the lab for a week, and by the way, don't forget the copay at the door. As for good advice, don't expect much from your eight-minute visit beyond "Don't do that again."

Many of my patients are pleasantly surprised to find that I'm young (in my thirties) and that I'm interested in hearing their worries about drugs, pregnancy, STDs, crash dieting, anxiety, stress, sexual performance, and other thorny issues. Unfortunately, these questions vexing people in my age group are not the ones I was trained to answer. Does Xanax take the edge off work-related stress? How bad is cocaine for you . . . *really*? Does weekend smoking cause cancer? These aren't easy questions, but after much time spent poring over the medical literature, and after interviewing many top specialists, I was able to find the information my patients were searching for. This book is the result.

Some people will look at this advice and suggest that *The Healthy*

Guide to Unhealthy Living will encourage bad habits, but I don't think that's the case. My patients will back me up on this: I tell them that they shouldn't make the unhealthy choices they make. But I also know that lectures saying "Don't have sex" and "Don't drink too much" are unlikely to register with people who think they're invincible. I don't advocate illegal behavior, but I don't judge my patients if they admit to it in my office. My job as a doctor is not to impose my values on my patients, but rather to learn about their lives and their health and give them the information to make their own—hopefully intelligent—choices. If a patient tells me she drinks a lot and wants to mitigate the damage, but isn't ready to quit her weekend binges, I'll tell her what she can do. If she trusts that I have her best interests in mind, she's more likely to listen when I tell her that she's better off cutting back.

If you work a sensible, nonstressful nine-to-five job; if you're in a monogamous relationship; if you abstain from smoking, drugs, and alcohol; and if you are completely content in life, this book is not for you.

But if you've been known to drink, smoke, hook up, work too hard, or eat fast food for six meals in a row, this book will help you manage your bad habits, and may change the way you see your choices.

While you can follow many of my suggestions on your own, others require prescription drugs that are available only through consultation with a doctor. The last chapter of this book will help you navigate the medical system and figure out how to partner with your doctor to ensure the best care. While going to the doctor is never fun, the anxiety of worrying about your health is worse. If this book does nothing else, I hope to convince young professionals that even if you haven't been a model patient when it comes to your health, you have nothing to lose from seeking help if you need it. Bad habits can be kicked, but it's tough to do so on your own. **None of the information in this book is meant to substitute for your own doctor's advice, so always consult your primary physician if you have questions about your health.**

A Note on Anonymity

Throughout the book, I use anecdotes to illustrate the lifestyles and medical problems that real people deal with. Many of my patients are high-profile individuals used to seeing their names in the newspapers, but like any patients, they are entitled to doctor-patient confidentiality. So while this book's anecdotes are based on true stories, all the identifying details, including names, have been changed.

One

Pushing the Limits

THE first time I saw a patient I'll call Mr. Stress, his nervous twitching and lack of eye contact brought to mind the terror I experienced at age sixteen when I tried to ask girls out on dates.

Mr. Stress was the new chief financial officer at a major company. He'd done several stints at smaller firms, and now had a shot at the big leagues. As he pored over his new company's financials, however, he realized that his predecessor had been fudging numbers for years. After the Enron debacle, he knew the stock market would not look favorably on accounting mistakes. Now he was left holding the bag for a correction that was bound to send the stock price tumbling.

He came into my office with symptoms that resembled a heart attack: chest pains, racing heartbeat, tingling in his fingertips. All of these had increased in intensity as his new job became more stressful. Now they were keeping him from getting his job done.

I figured out within the first few minutes that Mr. Stress's problem wasn't "medical," in the sense that cancer or AIDS are "medical." A lifestyle change, such as quitting his job and heading for the Bahamas, would have cleared up the twitching faster than any medication I could have given him.

But since he couldn't walk away from the problem, we had to deal with the very real physical effects of extreme anxiety on his body. If he was going to be able to think and work effectively, he had to put himself back in charge. We discussed his options, and decided to start him on Lexapro, an antidepressant with few side effects, and the tranquilizer Klonopin for anxiety. Within three visits, I could see a difference. The accounting figures hadn't magically corrected themselves, but he was a new man. No more twitching. No more slouching. He walked into the room like the confident executive he was. Once the symptoms of his anxiety were under control, *he* was in control again. Over the next six months, he managed to pull the company's books together and avert disaster. Indeed, once the crisis was over, he was able to stop taking his medications completely. Like many of my patients, Mr. Stress just needed a little help to steer through the rough patches of life.

• • •

While we don't all have accounting scandals to deal with, stress, depression, and anxiety affect everyone from executives to unemployed new college grads trying to make ends meet. Soon after I started practicing in New York, I learned that in the city that never sleeps, some people really never do. When the rent check is due but the money isn't there, when a promotion is just one big deal away, or when the general worries of too much work and too little time weigh on us, we need that extra push to stay in control.

Stress, anxiety, depression, lack of sleep, and the ability to concentrate have much to do with your health. But few people see their doctors about these so-called lifestyle issues. I talk with almost all my patients about the health issues that arise from pushing the limits, but usually not because the patient tells me he's been working until two A.M. for two weeks straight, or that he is terrified of making a presentation to his superiors.

Instead, he'll come in with nonspecific complaints: sleeplessness, a pounding or irregular heartbeat, chest pains, body aches, and fatigue. Or he'll have headaches that begin in the morning and increase during the day. Tests won't show anything physically wrong, but if I ask a few questions, and sit there and listen long enough, my patient will soon tell me that his brain is making him sick.

Adrenaline–a factor in many of these symptoms–is a tricky chemical. When lions chased our ancestors over African savannahs, the fight-or-flight response served a real purpose–it kept us from becoming cat chow. In this day and age, though, sweaty palms, a cracking voice, racing thoughts, and that dry-mouth feeling work against us. When you're at a job interview, or making a presentation on a million-dollar project, the adrenaline rush doesn't save you, it sinks you. And if it keeps you up at night, adrenaline just adds misery to discomfort.

Fortunately, we know a lot more about how the brain works than our lion-fleeing ancestors did. Several drugs and other techniques can help you beat the fight-or-flight response, stay awake, get to sleep, or make you feel better about your stressful life.

If you're lucky, you could try what one of my patients did. Emily was twenty-eight years old and had been working for an advertising agency for six years. During the past year, though, her increasing fatigue had started to hamper her functioning at the office. She'd sit through meetings, dazed, lost to the conversation and unable to connect with the other people in the room. Like many of my patients with stress-related symptoms, she had dull headaches that started in the morning and peaked in the midafternoon. She had lost interest in spending time with her friends and boyfriend. By the time she walked into my office, she was convinced she was suffering from depression. And she was right. But what she hadn't done was draw the connection between her symptoms and the stress she had heaped on herself over the last few years trying to outdo the competition in chasing after the shrinking advertising dollars in her field.

I often joke with my overstressed patients that they have two choices: Either pack up and head for the Virgin Islands, or consider a short trial of medication. In my experience, many professionals would rather take two pills a day and hone their performance at work than admit that the pressure is too much to bear and pack it in. If the guy across the hall is still at the top of his game, then *you* can't admit defeat.

For Emily, however, heading out to the beach was just what the doctor ordered. Rather than try to face her job with the help of a few drugs, she met with her HR department and explained that she needed to take a medical leave of absence. When she returned to my office armed with the volumes of requisite paperwork, I explained that there was no guarantee that the company would give her time off for headaches and fatigue. But to my surprise, her company accepted the diagnosis and granted her six months of leave to get her act together She jetted off to the islands for half a year of scuba diving and margaritas, and the next time I saw her she was a new person. Tan and relaxed, she was thankful for the time off and had a new perspective on life.

I wish more people, including myself, were able to take advantage of such opportunities to escape stress and enjoy life. But if that's not an option for you, read on for tips on how you and your doctor can help you stay healthy while you gain those extra advantages every ladder-climber needs.

Anxiety and Mood

Anxiety, stress, and depression are interlocking problems with similar symptoms and similar treatments. When a patient comes around to admitting her jitters or moodiness, we first talk about ways to calm one's emotions without drugs. My favorites include progressive muscle relaxation, self-hypnosis, meditation, biofeedback, exercise, and therapy.

Progressive Muscle Relaxation

Anxiety and stress contract your muscles. Your teeth clench, your hands shake, and your legs quiver. You can short-circuit that response by causing the contractions yourself, and then focusing on relaxing the major muscle groups.

Find a spot where people won't stare at you, then try this: contract, release, repeat. Start with the muscles that are easiest to see and focus on—the hands, arms, and legs. Contract these muscles, then let the tension go. After you are able to focus and see results, you can move to the muscles more responsible for your tension—the neck, back, and face. The contraction phase is important at first, because it's hard to learn to release a muscle you haven't contracted. But after a while you'll learn to release your tension without so pronounced a contraction, and then you can spend most of your time in the relaxing phase. Plan to spend at least one full minute, if not several minutes, on this technique.

Once you train yourself to focus only on the relaxation, you can repeat that focus in any situation. For instance, if you're an anxious traveler, try a "hands free" flight. Rather than grip the armrests, hold your hands in front of you and spread your fingers wide, focusing on relaxing all the muscles in your upper body. It's tough to stay stressed for long while doing this.

Self-hypnosis

Instead of clenching your muscles, start an inner monologue that promotes relaxation. Keep repeating to yourself "My body is relaxing," or "I am slowly letting go of the day's worries." Responses vary, but if you force yourself to slow down and focus on these words, you'll likely produce a few moments of calm.

You can create a similar calm feeling by focusing on a pleasant image. For instance, if you dread making presentations in front of crowds, spend some of your prep time envisioning a peaceful beach where you can speak freely. The more detailed the scene, the more you will find yourself focused on it, and therefore the less stressed you will be about your presentation. For this to work, of course, you'll need to prepare ahead of time, since you'll have to reserve those last few knuckle-cracking minutes for calm thoughts. But if stress was affecting your performance, those minutes will be time well spent.

Meditation

Meditation involves focusing solely on one thing—say, your breathing. Don't try to control it, just tune your mind to the rhythmic pattern. When other thoughts enter your brain—the mortgage, that presentation—replace them with "inhale, exhale." Meditation is slightly different from self-hypnosis because rather than focus on a scene, you focus on a rhythm that removes all thought and therefore all stress. Some of my more religious patients substitute prayer for meditation—communicating with the divine power they believe in, focusing solely on praying and nothing else. A few moments of prayer makes other concerns seem less pressing.

Clinical psychologists say you will need to work on any of these techniques—progressive muscle relaxation, self-hypnosis, and meditation—for at least two to four weeks before you begin to see consistent results. Mastering these techniques to the point where you experience relief quickly will take anywhere from six weeks to six months. So it's important to be patient. That's the bad news. The good news is that these exercises are easy to perform, have no nasty side effects, and don't cost a thing. So why not give them a try?

Biofeedback

When I use this technique in my office, I hook the patient to a machine that monitors heart rate, body temperature, and blood pressure—all body functions that are influenced by stress and anxiety. The patient sees his numbers reflected on a small monitor and works on changing them with focused meditation techniques such as those described above. By showing the patient instantly when the technique is working, biofeedback helps those most motivated by concrete results. If this sounds like you, then pick up the phone and ask your doctor to recommend a practitioner in your area who can help you get started.

Exercise

Some of my patients with gyms (and showers) in their offices swear by a twenty-minute sprint on the treadmill to blow off steam. Not only do you focus your mind on something other than work frustrations, your mood actually lifts as your heart starts pumping faster. It's hard to come out of a workout thinking "woe is me." If you can, work out during your lunch hour and eat at your desk later. If you don't have a gym, hike around the parking lot or do stair sprints (your coworkers won't notice, they take the elevator). If a midday workout's not possible, exercise before work in the morning. You can easily waste half an hour hunting for the perfect outfit or a clean shirt. For those suffering from mild depression or anxiety, exercise is a *much* better use of your time.

Therapy

Psychological counseling gets a bad rap ("No, how do you *really* feel about your mother?") and many of my patients are reluctant to try this option. They feel that as tough, competent individuals, they should be able to handle what life throws at them on their own. Even if they've lost weight and stopped showing up at work or enjoying life, somehow counseling is admitting defeat. But therapy isn't about defeat. The only thing that's defeatist is doing nothing about something that's bothering you.

For all the fear people have about therapy, the process isn't too frightening. Once you actually drag yourself through the door, the therapist will just start a conversation and ask, much as your doctor would, what brought you in. The conversation goes to whatever ails you: pressures at work, trouble with the spouse, or why you feel tired all the time. Think of the therapist as an objective ally—someone who will be even more focused on you than a close friend or family member might be, who will listen to what you say and how you say it, and help you solve your problems.

If you decide you'd like to try seeing a therapist, start by asking your doctor to recommend one in the area. If you're a member of a church, synagogue, or other house of worship, your minister will likely be able to recommend someone as well. Or talk to your friends; I'll bet at least one is seeing a therapist and will be glad to give you some insight. Just remember that it doesn't hurt to go. I've yet to have a patient who hasn't found therapy at least partially satisfying. In the worst case scenario, if you discover you hate it, you've just wasted the time it takes to watch *Divine Secrets of the Ya-Ya Sisterhood* or *Caddyshack* on DVD. So what?

I recommend people try whichever of these options they find appealing, but most important, I recommend that they try at least one of them. Even my patients who are apprehensive about holistic medicine have benefited from taking a jog or taking a few moments to breathe deeply. Think about it this way: There is no risk to trying meditation, for example, and there's a big possibility of feeling better.

I was reminded of that with one of my patients, John, who worked for a financial services firm known for making its young MBAs work twenty hours a day (with the consolation, of course, of salaries totaling several hundred grand a year). At age twenty-nine, John was charged with making weekly presentations to his firm's board of directors. He met with CEOs of publicly traded companies just as often. It's not easy for any young person to tell a sixty-year-old CEO how to run his company, but when this guy stepped up to the podium, he had severe heart racing, a trembling voice, and such profuse sweating that half his audience was tempted to dial 911.

John thought that the Xanax his friends had been taking would help. I prescribed the drug for him, but when he tried it, he felt too tired to present. We tried several other antianxiety medications; each in turn either didn't work or caused side effects that were worse than his original case of nerves. After several weeks, John decided to invest some time in counseling. The therapist we found for him used biofeedback to help him control his stress response. After a few months, without drugs, John became one of the best presenters in his firm.

Anxiety and Depression Medication

If you don't have success with these techniques, though, then it's time to talk with your doctor about medications that can relieve your anxiety with fewer drawbacks than self-medicating with alcohol, marijuana, or prescription drugs bummed from a friend. A bottle of wine may make you feel better, but alcohol is a dirty drug. You'll cause more anxieties for yourself by acting like a drunken idiot, and you won't improve whatever situation is causing your troubles by waking up with a hangover. Furthermore, excessive drinking causes more dependence issues than most other drugs. Chronic marijuana use leads to issues with job performance, memory, cognitive impairment, and even depression. Borrowed drugs can cause their own problems with side effects or drug interactions. While most of these drugs are safe when taken properly, you shouldn't take someone else's drugs.

When you see your doctor, she'll discuss a few drugs that can help. The first is Inderal (propranolol), which is in a class of medications called beta-blockers. Used primarily to lower blood pressure or to help treat an overactive thyroid, this short-acting medication blocks the receptors for adrenaline and smooths out the stress response. For most of my patients, it stops their hearts from pounding and their stomachs from churning when it comes time to make that speech in front of a crowd.

Inderal is not physically addictive, but it has a few side effects that make it not perfect for everyone. Some people complain of dizziness, nausea, or a slightly "not right" feeling. So I recommend you try it once before the big event to see whether you encounter these side effects. If the side effects don't bother you, great. If they are worse than you anticipated, then ask your doctor to try something else.

That something else is usually Klonopin (clonazepam), which I prescribed to Mr. Stress, or Xanax (alprazolam). These drugs are very similar to Valium, and work by triggering the GABA receptors in the brain. These are the same receptors that alcohol affects, and if you've ever had a few too many drinks, you know what they do—relax muscles, relieve inhibitions and anxiety, and induce sleep.

Klonopin and Xanax trigger the GABA receptors in a way that maximizes anxiety relief while minimizing sedation. In the right dose, they can calm your racing thoughts like a shot or two of Jim Beam, but without impairing cognition or coordination. Too much, and sedation takes hold—not a good prospect for a big interview or presentation. So just like Inderal, test-drive these drugs under your doctor's supervision before taking them when the side effects matter.

I'm often asked by patients whether these drugs are addictive, and unfortunately, the answer is not a simple yes or no. The word *addiction* has a different medical meaning than the way we use it in everyday conversation. Medically, "addiction" refers to a person exhibiting a craving for a substance that causes him to engage in self-destructive behavior to get that drug. It's more accurate to say that drugs such as caffeine or alcohol, or the medications used for anxiety, can create "tolerance." When a person builds up a tolerance to a drug, the brain creates more receptors for it, so that over time you need a higher dose to get the same results. The more coffee you drink, the more you'll need, over time, to get wired.

Anxiety drugs work the same way. That means that, over time, a patient taking Xanax might need 2 mg instead of one to get the same effect. This process usually takes months, and once you develop a tolerance, you'll need to taper down the drug rather than stop taking it entirely in order to avoid withdrawal symptoms.

However, people who don't take the drug daily for long periods of time won't develop a tolerance. If you only have an occasional cup of coffee, you won't get a headache if you don't have a cup within an hour of crawling out of bed. Anxiety drugs work the same way. So for short-term use, you don't need to worry much about dependence.

On the other hand, many patients and many doctors are concerned about dependence issues for long-term use of anxiety medicines, so it makes sense to consider drugs that can be taken daily and don't have any association with addiction. Antianxiety, antidepressant medications such as Prozac, Paxil, and Celexa or similar drugs such as Cymbalta or Effexor can fill this need. Anxiety and depression are closely related. Medicines that boost your mood can also soothe your jitters.

When your brain releases the neurotransmitters serotonin and norepinephrine, these chemicals bind to receptors that trigger feelings of calm and well-being. Antidepressants slow the brain's ability to process these chemicals. When the neurotransmitters aren't processed, they spend more time triggering those calm, well-being feelings. These drugs take a week or two to produce the full effect, so they're not great for a quick fix. However, if you need a lot of quick fixes, day after day, then antidepressants might be right for you.

Like antianxiety drugs, antidepressants smooth out emotions and curb symptoms of depression or anxiety–lack of enjoyment in life; insomnia or sleeping too much; lack of appetite or increased appetite; feelings of uselessness, agitation, or guilt–that can harm your performance. Everyone suffers from a few of these at times, and we're all prone to mood changes, but if these symptoms occur for more than a few days or weeks and interfere with your performance or relationships, they warrant discussion.

Unfortunately, antidepressant drugs carry a stigma for some people. If you feel that way and your doctor recommends you try one, keep this in mind. You can stop taking these drugs (after talking to your doctor) at any time, so don't think of it as a lifelong decision. You just need help for a little while until you figure out what lifestyle changes you can make to soothe your nerves and boost your mood. The most important thing is to do something. Anxiety and depression can be crippling, making you and everyone around you miserable. Deciding to talk to a doctor or therapist about them is difficult, but so is living with them. No harm comes from looking at all your options.

Sleep

Like the antianxiety drugs Xanax and Klonopin, most prescription sleep drugs trigger the GABA receptor. Unlike antianxiety drugs, sleep drugs focus on the sedation function–and put you out like a light. They don't work for everyone. One patient of mine had been through virtually every sleeping pill on the market. She's threatened to crack herself over the head with a frying pan to get to sleep. But usually these pills do the job.

Many prescription sleep drugs, however, are controlled substances with the potential to become habit-forming, and few insurance companies cover more than a few weeks of doses (partly so you won't use them as a crutch . . . and partly because the companies are cheap). So before you start relying on these drugs, consider this:

> Alcohol may help you fall asleep, but it won't help you stay asleep, and over time—especially when paired with nicotine and caffeine—it can contribute to insomnia.

A few glasses of wine will make you sleepy, but if you've ever passed out drunk, you know even twelve hours of sleep won't make you feel rested. All you're ready to do is sit in front of the TV with your hands embedded in a bag of chips.

While alcohol triggers the GABA receptors responsible for sedating you, there's a problem. As the alcohol wears off, your energy level rebounds as a surge of adrenaline kicks in, peaking when your blood alcohol level approaches zero. So if you've had four drinks, you're quite likely to wake up four hours later, usually sweating and with a headache. Couple that with stumbling out of bed to go to the bathroom and you'll have trouble getting back to sleep.

Then in the morning, when you need to be at work, and you're still not rested, you'll have several cups of coffee or smoke a few cigarettes to stay awake. While most people avoid coffee or a smoke right before bed, even daytime use of these common drugs can affect sleeping habits, since both caffeine and nicotine linger in the system. So you have a few more drinks to fall asleep. Then you wake up several hours later when your blood alcohol level falls. The rebound alertness is compounded by caffeine and nicotine.

Most of my patients with fatigue and insomnia are self-treating with alcohol and coffee. Each makes the effect of the other worse, and prevents the patient from being sleepy at night and awake during the day. Breaking this cycle of being sleepy only when you don't want to be is the first step to getting a good night of sleep.

> Over-the-counter sleep drugs say "Don't operate heavy machinery" on the package for a reason— they leave a wicked hangover.

Just about every OTC sleeping aid is an antihistamine, and many of my patients take drugs such as Benadryl (diphenhydramine) or Tylenol PM to help them fall asleep. Sure, they work, but they'll keep working long after the eight hours you hoped to sleep.

The goal of any insomnia treatment is to put you to sleep at night and keep you awake during the day. Antihistamines cause daytime drowsiness. So in the morning, you'll still be incredibly groggy. You'll have three cups of coffee so you won't drive off the road on the way to work. This excess caffeine contributes to the sleepless cycle described above.

Beyond Alcohol and Benadryl

Fortunately, alcohol and OTC drugs aren't the only options if you don't want to try prescription drugs. The key is to understand the physical forces that govern sleep.

People have circadian rhythms that drive their sleeping and waking cycles. These cycles run between twenty-four and twenty-seven hours, so they're not exactly aligned with the twenty-four-hour day. The body relies on external triggers to shift the sleep cycle to coordinate with the clock. These triggers include temperature, light, activity, and sex. Here's how to use these triggers to your advantage:

Avoid Long Naps

I've heard stories of guys catching fifteen-minute catnaps on the john in the men's room when they have to shut their eyes. It's not glamorous, but it will work. Anything more than twenty minutes, though, will disrupt your next sleep cycle.

Most adults in their twenties and thirties need seven hours of sleep a night. This tends to decrease as you get older, so that six hours a night might suffice a decade or two down the road. Some people need five, some need nine, but if you fall asleep within one minute of hitting the pillow, you're not getting enough sleep. You probably experience a period of general sleepiness eight hours after waking (when most people head for that afternoon cup of coffee). Instead of the coffee, try closing your office door for ten minutes and catching a quick nap. You won't interfere with your sleep cycle, and you won't go into deep REM sleep. Morning or evening naps, though, will just keep you awake longer at night.

Don't Oversleep

Try going to bed at the same time and waking up at the same time every day. Sunday nights are prime time for insomnia. In addition to dealing with the worries of the upcoming week, you probably woke up at noon. Your body isn't ready to go to sleep at eleven P.M.

Of course you're going to stay up later on Friday and Saturday nights than on Tuesday nights, but resist the temptation on Saturdays and Sundays to sleep more than an hour or two past your normal wake-up time if you want to sleep normally during the week.

Light Matters

Thousands of years of evolution have conditioned us to wake up when we see bright lights. Try to get some sunshine within an hour of awakening (or as soon as the sun comes up, if you've got the early shift during a Minnesota winter), and avoid bright lights during the evening or if you wake up in the middle of the night. Use a nightlight in the bathroom and don't stand there with the refrigerator door open. Those with real trouble functioning in the morning can consider buying a broad-spectrum UV sunlamp. These are available everywhere (do a Google search), and can mimic the beneficial effects of morning sun when used for thirty minutes daily.

Exercise

Exercise keeps your body's sleep cycle regular and can make you feel more relaxed and alert during the day. Get some exercise daily, but not too close to bedtime, when the adrenaline rush might keep you awake. Early afternoon is best, perhaps right after that ten-minute nap.

Watch the Temperature

Being too hot or too cold will keep you from sleeping–your body is programmed not to let down its guard if it worries you'll freeze or burn during the night—but being a little warm helps. Take a hot bath, drink a warm noncaffeinated beverage, or use a down comforter to feel cozy enough to dream.

Limit Caffeine, Alcohol, and Nicotine

Anything except a morning cup of coffee can affect sleep. I recommend no caffeine after ten A.M. Drink alcohol at happy hour or early evening, but not late at night if you have trouble sleeping. Move that after-dinner smoke (if you must) to after work, so you are nicotine-free by bedtime.

Nix the Stress

Don't look at the time. It will only upset you to see the numbers ticking past two . . . three . . . four A.M. Focus on relaxing, not sleeping. If you're anxious, take some time to focus on the problems that worry you and make a plan for what you will do tomorrow to address them. If you can't fix a problem, write your worries in a journal, punch the pillow, or talk to someone who cheers you up. You can also try a relaxation technique such as meditation or progressive muscle relaxation (pages 8–10).

Use the Bed Only for Sleeping and Sex

Spending a rainy afternoon reading in bed is nice, but if you do too many activities under the covers, your body will stop thinking "sleep" when it sees your pillow. Sex is the obvious exception to the "no activities" rule. For starters, the kitchen counter is unlikely to take over beds in the favorite sex spot department anytime soon, and sex makes many people (especially guys) sleepy. If you're one of the unfortunates who become restless after sex, then try to avoid sex right before sleep. Get up thirty minutes before you need to and go off to work with a bang. Your partner might be pleasantly surprised.

Realize You Won't Make Up a Sleep Deficit in a Night

If you can't sleep enough on a regular basis, don't expect to make it up all at once. The body remembers about a week of sleep. If you need seven hours but you consistently get six over a week, you build up a sleep deficit of seven hours in addition to what you usually need, so you'll need two to three days to make it up. Figure that into your schedule, and don't plan to recoup it all on Saturday night.

Try Melatonin or Other Herbal Remedies

The hormone melatonin peaks as you go to sleep and drops off as you wake. You can purchase a version of this hormone over the counter at drugstores or vitamin shops. Studies show that taking anywhere from 5 to 80 mg three to four hours before bedtime can help tell your body that it's time to go to sleep (the evidence isn't so strong for taking melatonin immediately before bedtime).

While melatonin won't cure a committed insomniac, it's easy to find, fairly cheap, has no real side effects if used sporadically, and you can stop using it at any time. So it's worth a shot. Some of my patients find melatonin useful for long plane flights. If you're flying to Europe (eastbound), take a dose around six P.M. as you're clearing security. You should fall asleep after the flight attendants clear dinner. Once you arrive, take another dose the next four nights a bit before bedtime so you won't wake up at three A.M.

Since the flight back to the United States (westbound) from Europe is during daylight hours, you won't need to sleep on the flight. But you can take a dose the next four nights before bedtime to make sure you fall asleep and don't wake up until morning.

The only other herbal medication that's been proven to work for insomnia is valerian root. Anywhere from 300 to 600 mg before bed can improve sleep, though you may need four weeks to see results, based on available research. Other herbal concoctions advertised as sleep aids—including chamomile, passionflower, lavender, catnip, and hops—work for some people, but I've not seen any data to back that up. There's no harm in trying them. Just don't expect miracles.

Some combination of all these methods works for many people. But even if some of the methods help, sleep triggers change, so one may stop working after a while. If that's the case, then it may be time to try prescription sleeping pills.

Rx Zzzzzz . . .

Three popular drugs, Sonata, Lunesta, and Ambien, all act quickly, and leave the body more quickly than, say, OTC antihistamines. Sonata lasts about four hours, Ambien six to eight, and Lunesta a little longer. If your problem is waking up in the middle of the night, take Ambien or Lunesta at bedtime rather than Sonata. However, if you don't take a sleeping pill before going to bed, and you wake up in the middle of the night, Sonata will put you back to sleep but won't leave you groggy when you need to wake up at seven A.M.

These drugs can also improve sleep after you've had a few drinks. They counteract the rebound effect when your blood alcohol level dips. Don't take them with more than two or three drinks—you will overdo it and make yourself too sluggish for safety. But for a moderate drinker, they can improve sleep and improve performance the next day.

Some patients report having trouble falling asleep without sleep drugs once they start taking them. But since these patients had trouble falling asleep before taking the drugs as well, it's hard to say that sleep drugs are responsible for the subsequent insomnia. Of course, never take sleeping pills when you are anywhere other than in bed (or in your airplane seat), and then stay there. If you do start wandering around after taking these medications, things can get dicey pretty quick. Erratic behavior, hallucinations, and amnesia are common. You can walk and talk for hours and then not remember a thing. One patient of mine took Ambien when he was having trouble sleeping in his Cancun hotel room on vacation. Then he decided that the party outside sounded like it was more fun than his bed. He has no idea how he ended up in the hotel lobby in his underwear, and I doubt he'll ever find out. Bottom line: Stay in bed. It also goes without saying that you shouldn't operate any vehicle or machinery while taking these pills.

Drugs such as Valium, Klonopin, and Xanax will also relax you, but they aren't as reliable for getting to sleep. That's why they are so effective for *daytime* anxiety.

Boredom and Fatigue

While some people's jobs keep them awake at night from stress and anxiety, there's a more common ailment plaguing the cubicle workers of today's world: boredom.

A first-year law associate sifts through court documents again, trying to push his way toward sixty billable hours a week. A consultant pores over a spreadsheet trying to figure out ways to save another penny on every widget. Some careers are only glamorous from the outside, and many of my patients devote their considerable creativity to devising ways to stay alert at white-collar sweatshop jobs that not only require long hours but are slowly boring them to death.

Caffeine is everyone's favorite stimulant. It also has some serious downsides. Too much coffee causes tremors and jitteriness, diarrhea, thirst, and indigestion. Caffeine destroys the stomach lining over time, and the tolerance it creates means that you soon need two pots of coffee a day to stay awake. There's a reason Starbucks can afford to open a shop on every corner. As far as drugs go, caffeine is right up there with nicotine in terms of getting you hooked.

One of my first patients, a thirty-year-old investment analyst, came to the office after her racing heart, chest pains, shortness of breath, jitters, and unsteadiness scared her into making an appointment. Her father had a history of early heart disease, so we did some tests.

An electrocardiogram, exercise stress test, and echocardiogram were all negative. I had her come to the office to go over the results. At this point, she confessed that she was sleeping two or three hours a night and drinking cappuccinos nonstop to stay awake and somewhat functional. Add in an after-work glass of wine here and there to relax, and she was about as drugged as you can get without a prescription.

All we had to do was take her off the caffeine and have her inform the office—doctor's orders—that she had to get more sleep, and the problem went away. In fact, her performance improved as she started working fewer hours. As one of my business school professors put it, we all need a few days here and there to sharpen our axes.

Caffeine's not the only over-the-counter stimulant that can cause problems; many people have gotten themselves into trouble using ephedrine to stay alert. This drug isn't commonly available anymore after investigators linked it with several deaths and the FDA banned ephedra (the herbal substance containing ephedrine), but it still gets around.

One of my patients came in with a cold, but an exam found that his blood pressure was an eye-popping 190/120 (about twice normal). His heart rate (over 120) was also twice what it should have been for someone whose most strenuous exertion in the previous five minutes was leafing through a magazine. Turns out he had just popped a couple ephedrine tabs before coming into the office and we had a ringside seat to watch the effects.

My recommendation: Don't take this drug. There are easier ways to give yourself a lift, and without the risk of having a coronary.

One safer way to improve your focus is to follow treatments designed for attention deficit disorder (ADD). While figuring out whether you have ADD or whether your job just stinks is subjective (see below), some adults so obviously have ADD, they practically have it tattooed on their foreheads. ADD medication drastically improves these people's lives.

Jackie, a thirty-something patient of mine, worked as an administrative assistant. After introducing herself at her first visit, she kicked her shoes across the room, and then hopped on and off the scale—three times. Then she talked a mile a minute about her sushi-ordering habits. Then she had a seat. Then she stood up. Then she had a seat. Then she switched, with no transition, from talking about sushi to recounting something about the office. Then she curled into the fetal position on the exam table.

As we talked, Jackie told me she'd been in three relationships in the past year, and had lived with two of these men. She was trying to change jobs, too, her fifth time in as many years.

I wasn't surprised to hear that other doctors had prescribed antidepressants—a common approach for patients who are worried about their lives. The drugs didn't work; Jackie would be the first to tell you she wasn't depressed. We agreed that she should try taking Ritalin, and sure enough, a few weeks later she called to tell me she was no longer running a relay race between the watercooler, the copier, and the window every fifteen minutes.

While Jackie's lack of focus cried out for a diagnosis of and treatment for ADD, many people have more subtle symptoms. Anything from poor concentration at the office, to trouble focusing, lack of energy, or general fatigue can be a symptom of attention deficit disorder. Here are the criteria your doctor will use for making a diagnosis:

MEDICAL CRITERIA FOR ADD

Six or more of the following, experienced *often*

- Inattention to details and making careless mistakes
- Difficulty organizing things
- Difficulty paying attention
- Avoiding tasks requiring sustained concentration
- Appearing not to listen
- Getting easily distracted
- Losing things
- Being forgetful
- Abandoning tasks in the middle

FOR HYPERACTIVITY

Six or more of the following, experienced *often*

- Impulsiveness
- Blurting out answers before the question is finished
- Fidgeting
- Have difficulty waiting your turn
- Being unable to stay seated
- Inappropriate running or climbing
- Being "always on the go"

- Restlessness
- Have difficulty engaging in quiet leisure activities
- Talking excessively
- Interrupting or intruding on others

A diagnosis requires that these symptoms must have persisted for six months or longer, be more frequent and severe than is normal for a person of that age, have begun before age seven, cause some impairment in two or more settings such as at school or at work, and be separate from any other mental disorders the person may have.

Clinical research shows that adults with ADD have problems keeping a job, are attracted to stimulating but risky professions, have trouble maintaining relationships, fail to clean or cook for themselves regularly, can't keep appointments, engage in dangerous driving, and enjoy stimulating sports for leisure.

By now, alert readers are rolling their eyes at these detailed–but broad–medical criteria. Who doesn't have difficulty keeping all their appointments? I don't know anyone who's single who cooks and cleans for him- or herself regularly. And let's not get started on having trouble focusing at work. If your job involves crunching numbers on a spreadsheet from nine A.M. to two A.M. every day of the week, none of these symptoms have much to do with ADD/ADHD, but have everything to do with the fact that your job requires more attention than humans were designed for.

If this describes you, and you're finding you just can't keep functioning, you have a choice. You can quit your job, or you can consider treatments–beyond caffeine–that enhance alertness and concentration. Several stimulants, including Concerta, Ritalin, Dexadrine, and Provigil, can improve your work performance. These drugs affect the brain in slightly different ways, but all of them can turn an adult who can't go five minutes at his cubicle without bidding on Grateful Dead memorabilia on eBay into a high-octane workaholic.

Many adults can benefit from occasional use of these drugs.

There are few downsides to a trial, and the effects show within the first few doses. Sure, some people use these drugs for what I'd say aren't the world's best reasons. A pharmaceutical sales rep I know takes Ritalin before going to the gym because it gives him extra energy without the scary side effects of ephedrine. One woman told me she takes ADD medications before she goes out on Friday nights because they allow her to stay out late without indulging in cocaine and other harmful drugs. Most people, though, use them only on occasion—when a huge project is due the next morning and caffeine will make them too jittery to perform. If you've been fueling your energy and your waistline with Starbucks and Krispy Kreme, a different tactic might be worth a try.

A Note on Prescriptions

I live in the real world. I know it's easy to find any of the drugs I list in this chapter without setting foot in a doctor's office. But because of the overlapping symptoms of stress, anxiety, depression, and attention deficit disorder, you should speak with your physician first about your specific complaints before taking any pills that you've scrounged up from your friend's medicine closet or off the Internet.

Sure, it's unlikely that any young, healthy person would suffer serious complications from these medications, but that's beside the point. You want to make sure you're getting the best possible treatment. You'll need some guidance to decide whether Klonopin, for example, or Provigil is right for your situation. Your doctor can also help you combine drugs with therapy to pack a double whammy in improving your mood and focus.

Climbing the career ladder is tough. Stress, anxiety, depression, and sleeplessness can keep all of us from reaching our goals. Fortunately, many treatments can help you regain your edge until you can make the healthy changes in your lifestyle that will put your cool, collected self back in charge.

Two

Everyday Vices: Alcohol and Tobacco

I STARTED SMOKING in medical school, ironic as that sounds.

In med school, we doctors-to-be heard over and over again how bad smoking was for you. We must not have been listening, though, because I've never seen so many smokers in my life. Every time we had five minutes to spare someone was slapping shut the anatomy book and slipping out for a smoke. Truth is, nicotine is an effective stimulant, and cigarettes can make ten hours of studying seem like nine.

My smoking habit only got worse during my internship in Boston. No matter what hospitals tell you, interns and residents still work eighty to a hundred hours a week, often in thirty-six-hour shifts. I had been a half-pack-a-day social smoker during medical school, but in the hospital, a half-pack turned into a full pack as my stress level rose. A smoke break gave a momentary respite from the day, and holding the cigarette—and taking a drag and feeling the nicotine calm my nerves—was a pleasure unmatched by anything we were seeing at the hospital.

My time as a smoker now helps me understand why many of the smart professionals I see in my office—people who *know* how bad smoking is for them, long term—cling to the habit. Nicotine wakes you up as quickly as coffee does, but unlike coffee, a cigarette forces you outside, away from your desk. Nicotine gives you a momentary buzz, just like alcohol, only smoking a cigarette won't impair your performance, and you can smoke before noon. With twenty cigarettes in a pack, waving one around and asking "Smoke break?" is a sure way to grab at least one or two people to join you. So smoking is a social experience as well.

Before I smoked, I never understood the gaggles of men and women outside their office buildings in the rain or snow, clustered over their cigarettes. Once I started smoking, however, those gaggles became not evidence of a pathetic addiction, but quick fifteen-minute vacations with friends. Smoking calms your nerves quickly, gets you some fresh air, then gets you back inside by the time the butt stops smoldering in the ashtray.

Most of us don't get enough vacation time, and so, the more you work, the more appealing smoking becomes. Fortunately for my health, I moved to San Diego after I finished my stint in Boston and started working a more sensible sixty-hour week. Miraculously, my desire to smoke faded with my memories of snowy weather. I took up surfing and trained for a marathon. I was so relaxed I broke my cigarette habit without even trying.

Back on the East Coast now, I've learned that New York City is more like Boston than San Diego. Here, I've seen my patients smoking to slog through their hundred-hour workweeks in Gotham's white-collar sweatshops. I've heard of offices where it's easier to calculate the number of hours people *don't* work. Couple that stress with a NYC party scene that centers around a few drinks after work, drinks over dinner, and drinks to end the night, and you can imagine how many times per week I encounter the question "How bad are smoking and drinking for me, *really?*"

Alcohol and nicotine are drugs like any other. Unlike heroin, though, if you follow a few social rules (go outside to smoke, no martinis at business lunches, and don't act obviously drunk) you can partake of these vices in polite company without being judged too harshly. So we indulge in alcohol and smoking more often than we probably should. If it's been a bad week, *way* more often than we probably should.

The bad news is that, no matter what you do, too much alcohol will give you a hangover and can damage the liver and pancreas, among other things. Too much smoking will raise your risk of heart disease and lung cancer. Together, the combination puts you at increased risk of esophageal cancer.

The good news is that neither of these vices is all that harmful in moderation. A bit of alcohol, in fact, is good for you. Tobacco's serious health effects can be mitigated by a few puffs of risk management on the way to quitting. So here's to these everyday vices, and to enjoying the pleasure while minimizing the pain.

Vice 1: Tobacco

Of my twenty- and thirty-something clients, about half are social smokers. We know that smoking a pack a day is a sure way to increase your risk of heart disease, strokes, or cancer, but what's less clear is whether smoking two cigarettes every Friday night when you are out for drinks will harm your health as well. We all know at least one geezer who smokes like a chimney and drinks like a fish, and at age ninety-five is still buying ladies drinks and offering to light their cigarettes. Is he the exception or the rule?

Unfortunately, the stats on cigarettes are stark. Even one puff is enough to temporarily damage lung function. In the long term, the consequences of smoking can be tragic.

Fortunately, your body has a remarkable ability to heal itself. So here's a little secret you won't see in the surgeon general's warning. Unless you're phenomenally unlucky, you can smoke socially in your twenties and live to tell about it in your seventies. The trick is quitting early—and successfully.

This isn't as easy as it sounds. If you could quit on a whim, there wouldn't be as much fuss about smoking as there is. But the simple truth is that smoking *for a little while* is unlikely to put you at risk for the most serious health problems.

How Tobacco Affects Your Body

The warnings on cigarette packs are based on well-tested science. Long-term studies have found that smokers have a higher risk of lung cancer, a higher risk of dying of heart attacks, and in fact die, overall, ten years younger than their nonsmoking counterparts. Tobacco damages a variety of body parts, including . . .

. . . the Heart and Brain

Strokes and heart attacks are caused by blockages in the small vessels leading to the brain and heart. Cholesterol plaques can build up in these vessels and then rupture. The cholesterol in the plaque spills into the vessel, causing a blood clot that blocks the artery that supplies blood to the organ. Block the path to the heart, you get a heart attack; block the path to the brain, you get a stroke.

Many lifestyle factors such as poor diet or lack of exercise cause plaque buildup, but cigarettes speed the process. When you take a puff, the nicotine in a cigarette immediately increases your heart rate and blood pressure. The drug inflames and constricts the small arteries that feed the heart and brain, making it more difficult for blood to deliver oxygen to these organs, and speeding plaque formation as well.

Tobacco smoke also increases your chance of blockages by making your platelets stickier. Platelets are little particles that float in the bloodstream until they find a rupture in the smooth surface of a vessel wall. When they encounter a rupture, they adhere and form a clot. Normally, this is a good thing; the clots platelets form on cuts and scrapes keep you from bleeding profusely. However, when cigarette smoke causes platelets to become extra sticky, there is an increased risk of clots forming in your bloodstream. Combine these clots with the cholesterol plaques cigarettes help form in the arteries, and you have a greater risk of heart attack or stroke. This is the reason doctors recommend an aspirin a day; the aspirin makes platelets *less* sticky and therefore reduces the risk.

. . . the Lungs

Cigarettes not only deposit tar and other chemicals in the lungs, they also impair the normal lung cleaning process. Your upper airways are lined with small hairs, or cilia, that move phlegm and particles up and out, leaving your lungs free of obstructions. One puff on a cigarette paralyzes these tiny hairs. If one puff or a few puffs is all you take, the conveyor belt will restart soon enough; however, if you are smoking daily, these hairs become permanently damaged and cease to be able to clear toxins from the lungs.

Cigarette smoking also damages your lungs by turning you into a "blue bloater" or a "pink puffer," to use the affectionate medical nicknames. Blue bloaters suffer from inflammation in the upper airways, a condition known as chronic obstructive pulmonary disease, or COPD. Their lungs act like those of an asthmatic. The airways constrict, trapping air in the lungs and making it difficult to breathe. The chest enlarges, and the skin takes on a mottled bluish tinge because the blood lacks oxygen. These patients need one or more types of oral or inhaled medications to improve breathing, and generally move slowly, taking long deep breaths to try to get air past the tight airways.

Pink puffers suffer from emphysema. In these patients, cigarette smoke has eroded the delicate areas of the lung that absorb oxygen from the air and transmit it to the bloodstream. The lungs can move air in and out, but the oxygen can't get into the body where you need it. These people tend to be thin, breathing rapidly to move air in and out quickly, and likely will need oxygen therapy at some point because the condition isn't reversible.

An invincible twenty-year-old can't conceive of being strapped to an oxygen tank when she's sixty, though, so many people still smoke, despite the warnings. Some of my patients *do* absorb the warnings, but like the buzz enough to ignore them. Many of these folks try to mitigate their risks by chewing tobacco or smoking cigars instead of puffing cigarettes. They're onto something . . . sort of.

Chewing Tobacco

I learned early in my medical career not to take a patient's habits for granted. As I was taught in med school, I always asked patients about cigarette smoking. I assumed that my patients understood that to mean they should tell me about any other tobacco habits, but . . . Real world lesson number one: Never assume anything. One young trader who came to my office denied smoking, but after I let the subject go he added that he would dip chewing tobacco at his desk all day long. Apparently his colleagues didn't mind if he used his coffee cup as a spittoon as long as he didn't confuse it with anyone else's. Since one in twenty Americans uses smokeless tobacco, and the rate is higher in the Southeast, I've become better at picking up this habit in my patients who are Dixie transplants.

Dipping tobacco, in theory, should raise your risk of gum and oral cancers, since the carcinogens in the tobacco seep right into the skin instead of entering the body through the lungs. Like most twenty-somethings, my patient couldn't have cared less about dying of heart disease at age fifty-five. However, since gum and oral cancers are usually caught early, death isn't the issue. For the vain, these cancers invite a worse prospect–multiple surgeries to remove the tumors, which in some cases lead to removal of the entire jaw. While death rarely deters people from their unhealthy activities, the thought of reaching age thirty without a lower jaw is a bit more sobering.

That's the bad news on dipping. The good news is that there have been tons of studies on oral cancers and dipping tobacco, and a consensus is hard to come by. The Scandinavians say there's no association, the Indians say there's a strong association, and the American studies don't show anything. Doctors find only a few thousand cases of oral cancer every year, so with numbers that small it's tough to prove any causal links. While it is likely that chewing tobacco increases your risk of getting an oral cancer, it is still unlikely to happen to you, specifically, and in general the overall risk of death is lower for dipping than smoking tobacco (that's how lethal lung cancer is). In fact, some experts have advocated switching to chewing tobacco as a way to stop smoking, although I doubt these experts have ever had to work with someone who carries a spittoon to the office. Nor have they been romantically involved with such a person. A word of advice to men who dip: Women consider spitting right up there with passing gas in public on the list of Things That Gross You Out So Much You Won't Sleep with Someone.

If you do decide to chew tobacco, or are already chewing, your best bet is to schedule a semiannual checkup with your regular doctor and an ear, nose, and throat specialist to make sure you aren't developing any precancerous lesions. This will limit your risk while you work on kicking the habit, and give your doctor a chance to identify and remove any precancerous lesions *before* they require major, jaw-removing surgery.

Cigars

Cigars are increasingly popular, even among doctors, and for good reasons. While *The New England Journal of Medicine* stopped shy of *recommending* cigar smoking, a major study published in 1999 failed to draw a connection between cancer and occasional cigar smoking. People who smoked less than five cigars a day had a slightly higher risk of developing heart disease, but not a significantly higher risk of developing any type of cancer, including lung and oral cancers. Even the incidence of heart disease in this group was relatively low—during the ten years of the study, the risk of heart disease for cigar smokers versus nonsmokers was 15.4 percent versus 13.7 percent, less than an extra 2 percent.

Two percent is a slight risk, but the important word here is *slight,* and the risk would not apply to the average cigar smoker who indulges a few times per week at most. Even the study's authors stopped shy of generalizing the results to occasional cigar smokers. For those of you smoking more than five cigars a day, the numbers don't crunch in your favor, but I'll trust that your friends' disgust at visiting an apartment that resembles a poorly ventilated smokehouse will moderate your habit soon.

Quitting

If you smoke, the occasional cigar makes a good substitute for a cigarette habit, if you can manage the transition. But even if you can't, here's some good news about smoking.

I promised you the opportunity to look cool in your twenties and still live to your seventies, and here's how. Smoking is bad for you, but it doesn't matter how much you smoke, or when you start. *Quitting by the time you are thirty mitigates almost all the damage.*

Smokers don't generally experience an elevated risk of dying from cancer, emphysema, or heart attacks until they turn fifty. Until then, from a health perspective, smokers and nonsmokers look a lot alike. After fifty, though, the difference is clear. In fact, smoking for thirty years takes, on average, ten years off your life. But your body has a remarkable ability to heal itself. A fifty-year longitudinal study of British doctors who smoked found quitting early is almost the same as not smoking at all.

This is why I've never harped on endlessly to my twenty-five-year-old patients on the dangers of smoking. What's the point? Anyone who doesn't live in a Philip Morris ad knows that smoking is bad for you, and we all want to live as long and as healthfully as we can. It's just a reality that smoking appeals to some people and they get hooked, as I once was, and not everyone is ready to quit.

One of the keys to quitting successfully is mental readiness. So what I do is ask my patients to plan a target date for *beginning* to think about quitting. Once the decision to quit has been made, we can forge a quit plan with a high likelihood of success.

I'm continually and pleasantly surprised that most smokers, while not ready to quit today, do want to quit eventually. With younger patients, I give them these stats, then let them know that their target is quitting by age thirty.

For those on the north side of thirty, it still isn't too late; every year of smoking works against you, but the effect doesn't escalate until you hit your forties. Smokers live ten years less than nonsmokers on average, but quitting by age thirty, forty, or fifty gives you back ten, nine, or six years, respectively. So it's never too late to quit and see increased longevity. I can't promise that if you stop smoking when you're fifty, you won't still suffer some lung and heart effects, but you will live longer.

It's not easy giving up cigarettes. If it were, I could tell you to puff away and give me a call when you turn thirty, but I can't. It's very difficult for anyone who smokes more than a few cigarettes a week to give up the habit. That's how cigarette companies make their boatloads of cash. But it can be done. The key is being mentally ready, and planning ahead.

The Nitty-gritty of Quitting

Every January, thousands of folks make New Year's resolutions to stop smoking, and by February 1, most of these people have fallen off the wagon. It's understandable. Cigarettes are addictive, and the day you quit you start suffering withdrawal symptoms including cravings, moodiness, insomnia, irritability, frustration, anger, anxiety, restlessness, and increased appetite. These are enough to test the resolve of any quitter. Overnight you go from a relaxed, friendly person who's up for a smoke break to a bitchy, irritable whiner who's gaining pounds by the minute. Quitters can expect to gain six to seven pounds on average once they stop smoking, thus sabotaging another frequent New Year's resolution. I'll save you the trouble right now: You won't lose weight and stop smoking in the same year.

In fact, the stats on quitting are grim even if you aren't trying to lose weight at the same time. Without medication, and without making some smart behavioral choices, you have only a 19 percent chance of success after seven weeks, and only a 12 percent chance of remaining smoke-free after a year.

Most people think it's the nicotine in cigarettes that lures them back for a smoke after a shot at quitting, but this is only half the story.

There are two mechanisms behind the impulse to continue smoking: the physical dependence on nicotine, and the behavioral dependence on grabbing a cigarette. Both are working to keep you hooked.

Nicotine is an addictive drug, which in medicine has a specific meaning. The brain creates nicotine receptors in response to added doses of the drug. Your brain knows that the drug is making you wired, but your brain finds running around wired all day tedious; therefore, it creates more and more nicotine receptors to take the drug out of circulation.

Unfortunately, unlike your brain, you *do* plan to stay wired on nicotine. So you react to the increased number of receptors by smoking more to get the same buzz. This cycle continues until you really do need a pack a day just to feel the same way you did the day *before* your first cigarette. You'll do some crazy things—including hunting around in your trash can for a cigarette if you've thrown them out because you're trying to quit—to get your fix.

Once you're smoking that much, your brain prompts you to keep the dose coming. Miss a dose, and you start experiencing withdrawal symptoms in proportion to how much of a hit you usually take.

Of course, your brain can adjust to the absence of an addictive drug. If you smoke a few cigarettes per day, and you stop smoking, you'll be intolerable to be around for the first twenty-four hours. But you'll be a lot less grouchy a few days in, and by the one-week mark you'll be addiction-free. This process takes different amounts of time for different people. If you smoke a lot, your withdrawal symptoms will be more severe and persistent, but they will go away in a matter of days or at most a few weeks.

Given this timeline, you can only blame the nicotine cravings if you relapse within the first few days or so after quitting. Most people making a serious quit attempt don't relapse so soon. The relapse occurs weeks later when you get a bad job review, your boyfriend picks a fight, or you're sitting outside a restaurant waiting for a friend who has a habit of being late.

You see, it's not only the physical dependence on cigarettes that hurts your chances of quitting, it's the behavioral dependence. For most smokers, smoking is a way to pass the time and relax. It lets you hop up from your desk for a ten-minute break during a stressful day with an excuse all your coworkers understand. Smoking gives you something to do when there is nothing to do. Check out any solitary person hanging out at a bar. The cigarette-less person appears to be waiting for someone, impatient and uncomfortable; the smoker is quietly enjoying his cigarette, anything else is an afterthought. After years of filling downtime by lighting up, it's tough to go back to that empty space. There are very few drugs that have been shown to help with this behavioral part of the habit, though many have been tried. Plenty of people try hypnosis or acupuncture, too, though neither of these has been proven, consistently, to help you stay off.

Because nicotine addiction is only half the problem, I rarely recommend nicotine gum or patches for anyone smoking less than a pack a day, despite some good data that nicotine replacement products help smokers quit. None of my patients quit and then relapse after two days. That's just missing a cigarette, not quitting. Sheer willpower can pull you through those first few days until you're no longer physically addicted. In fact, those are the easy days, because you're still committed to quitting. If you're committed, why extend your dependence any longer than you need to? It's the behavioral aspect you have to work on, or else you'll be bumming a friend's cigarette three weeks later, and that first week of discomfort and bad temper will have been for naught.

There's no secret to quitting. It's like running a marathon. It's going to hurt, and you're going to have to tough it out. Mastering one's mind is never easy. But you can make it easier with the following plan:

1. **Commit to quit.** I've seen people express a mild interest in quitting should nothing more interesting be happening in their lives, or mention offhand that they want to be able to smoke on vacation next month. An attitude like this will guarantee failure. Quitting is a big step, and one that should be taken seriously. Anyone who is ambivalent about quitting will have a much lower likelihood of success than someone who means to stop smoking for good.

   There are four stages in the quitting process:

   - precontemplation
   - contemplation
   - action
   - maintenance

   During the precontemplation phase, the smoker doesn't have any intention of quitting, and is merrily puffing away.

At this time, it's my job to gently push into contemplation, where the smoker is actively considering quitting. Then the real action can take place.

2. **Put yourself in an environment that does not encourage smoking.** You should join with your spouse or lover to quit together, and plan your social life based on your decision to quit, not the other way around. Too many people don't prepare to quit, figuring they can dive right in without thought. Unfortunately, most of these people relapse the first time a friend lights up in front of them. For this reason, I encourage patients to adopt the patterns of a non-smoker well before quitting. Make your home smoke-free. Put all the ashtrays outside. Ask your friends for support, and if they can't quit with you, put some distance between you and their bad habits.

3. **Pick a quit date.** We aren't going to taper down. This is cold turkey. Pick a date a few days or weeks into the future, and gear up for it by marking it in red on your calendar. Remember that the quit date can't be at a stressful time, such as in the same week as an annual performance review.

4. **Maximize your chances of success.** Find coping mechanisms to reduce your risk of relapse. I recommend that most of my patients take bupropion, a generic antidepressant marketed under the trade names Wellbutrin and Zyban. These drugs increase levels of dopamine and norepinephrine in the brain. These chemicals increase energy while decreasing cravings for everything, including food and cigarettes. A few folks can't take these drugs, including those with seizure disorders or stubborn hypertension. Also, a few people stop taking Wellbutrin or Zyban because of side effects including insomnia and jitteriness. For most people, though, bupropion can *double* the chance of quitting while curbing cravings and *halving* weight gain. Twice the benefits and half the weight gain–that's not bad.

If you are going to use these medications to increase your likelihood of success, you should begin taking the pills at least a week or two before the quit date so they have time to take effect. You can continue taking your pills for the first few months of quitting until you're sure you're past your cravings. The usual dose for smoking cessation is 150 mg, twice a day.

5. **Quit.** Now it's time to take the plunge. On your quit date, wake up and throw the cigarettes away. Not in your kitchen trash can, where you can dig them out. We're talking in a Dumpster two miles from your home. Go ahead and drive there and perhaps say a little requiem for the six dollars you spent on each pack. Now you are an official nonsmoker. The first few days are going to be rough, but you'll pull through. Bupropion will reduce your cravings, and your headaches and irritability will go away in a few days. Get rid of any smoking accessories (such as lighters and ashtrays) you still have around, and remember, *no cheating*. The quit date starts at midnight, so make sure you stick to that deadline (no four A.M. cigarette to bend the rules).

6. **Battle the relapse urge.** For the rest of your life, or until you are completely beyond any desire for tobacco, you'll have to ward off the temptation to pick up a cigarette. Avoid any situations where you'd be around smokers and cigarettes; find a contact person—a lover, friend, relative, or your doctor—who will be your first call if you start to think about smoking again. I've talked numerous people out of cigarettes on a Friday night. You're going to need some people who can support you, and they should know that you are using them for this reason (so they won't be annoyed when you keep calling).

7. **Exercise.** You should be doing this anyway, but an exercise program is a perfect complement to quitting. You ward off weight gain, and you take advantage of your

lungs' newfound health. My personal triumph over cigarettes came with my preparation for the Rock 'n' Roll Marathon in San Diego. The exuberance that comes from setting a new personal best time is a great substitute for a cigarette. Also, you can't help but feel a little silly lighting up after a ten-mile training run. Halfway into my training I quit without even trying.

8. Unfortunately, there is no last step. This is a lifetime decision, so plan to keep up your maintenance program indefinitely. Quitting gets easier as time goes by. Be sure to celebrate each milestone (first day, first week, first month, first year smoke-free) with something you'd enjoy as much as a cigarette.

While studies show that only 12 percent of quitters are smoke-free a year later, my own experience gives me greater confidence in people's ability to kick the habit when they truly want to. About 70 percent of my patients who want to quit smoking have done so successfully using the above techniques. So if you've been thinking about quitting, why not talk with your doctor and some friends about taking the plunge?

Vice 2: Alcohol

Since bar-hopping is New York's official sport, I can't tell you how often alcohol issues come up in my office. In fact, most of the minor accidents and injuries I see are somehow linked to drinking. Falling down the stairs is a classic. One of my patients was making her dramatic entrance into the New York social scene at the housewarming party of a celebrity's rooftop duplex. After three martinis, she missed the first step and tumbled head over heels the entire way down the stairwell, cutting her party time about three hours short.

Another one of my patients was out for a night on the town and failed to realize the dance floor was three steps down from the bar.

Not only did she not feel the fall, but she partied the rest of the night away in style. Monday morning, she came into my office with her left elbow swollen to the size of a grapefruit, and bruising from her wrist to the shoulder. The only way she made it through the night without her friends dragging her to the emergency room is that they were as tanked as she was.

Drunk stories are a lot less funny in the sober light of a doctor's office, so after a sheepish laugh, my patients bring the conversation around to the question: How much is too much? If you fall down the stairs and dislocate your shoulder after three martinis, then three martinis is your answer. But the good news is that drinking, unlike drinking to excess, is not necessarily a bad thing.

In fact, the medical data show that one of the best things you can do to improve your health and longevity, besides eating well and exercising, is to start drinking. Cardiovascular disease is the primary cause of death in most Western cultures, and a drink or two a day improves cholesterol profiles and reduces the risk of heart disease, stroke, and overall mortality. Many of my patients with low HDL (the good cholesterol) numbers are ecstatic to hear that my first recommendation to them is to start drinking one or two alcoholic beverages a day. Whether it's a scotch on the rocks or a beer with dinner, any alcohol will do. A shot of liquor, a glass of wine, and a bottle of beer all have the same amount of alcohol in them, and it's no coincidence that they're served in that fashion. There are some schools of thought that claim red wine is best, and red wine does have some antioxidants not found in other types of alcohol, but the cold hard facts support *all* alcohol, not just wine.

Before you toast away, though, this trend reverses at more than two drinks a day, since the damage to the brain and liver, not to mention your coordination, overrides the beneficial effects on the heart.

Right now I can picture the math whizzes out there cranking the numbers. Two drinks a day is fourteen drinks a week. So if you're sober Sunday through Thursday then guzzle seven drinks on Friday and Saturday, does this put you in the heart-healthy zone?

While the math may be right, the science isn't. Concentrating that two-drink average on one or two days is not the same thing as having a nightly glass of wine with dinner. Binge drinking is a separate category, and there all bets are off.

Binge drinking raises blood pressure, thus offsetting the cardiovascular benefits of moderate drinking. Binge drinking is also associated with impaired cognition, fatigue, poor coordination, and liver damage, not to mention high-risk sexual activity, drunk driving, and wicked hangovers.

Chronic drinking also depletes the body of thiamine (B_1) reserves. This can affect the nervous system, causing tremors, impaired coordination, and short-term memory loss. You may not notice these symptoms at first, but most binge drinkers will experience one or more episodes of poor functioning at some point.

Women (and some unlucky men) face an additional downside to heavy drinking. Alcohol has been linked to breast cancer, with each drink per day giving you approximately a 10 percent increase in the likelihood of developing the disease. The good news is that taking 1 mg of folate daily may offset the higher risk. Any woman of childbearing age should be taking this supplement anyway—deficiencies in folic acid are a primary cause of neural tube birth defects. (Most vitamins, especially prenatal ones, contain folic acid. Check the label to be sure.)

Aside from the blood pressure, breast cancer, and thiamine issues, too much alcohol just screws with your body, period. You don't need a doctor to tell you that. Volunteer in a soup kitchen sometime and see the health problems people with long-term substance abuse issues develop.

A few binges, on the other hand, do not a wino make. You have to consume about eight drinks a day for four or more years to cause permanent liver damage. Even during college, it's tough to maintain that kind of volume. Provided a friend is looking out for you and your car keys, and provided you don't really overdo it and wind up with acute alcohol poisoning or liver failure, the worst you'll suffer from the occasional binge is a lot of moaning the next morning that you'll never drink again.

As with most things in life, *moderation is key.*

Alcohol 101

Alcohol is water soluble and absorbed quickly by the body. About 20 percent of what you drink is processed in the stomach, and the rest enters your bloodstream through the gut, about thirty to sixty minutes after ingestion.

Cells that line the gastrointestinal tract contain alcohol dehydrogenase, which converts alcohol to acetaldehyde and then to acetate via yet another enzyme, aldehyde dehydrogenase. Acetate can be used as energy or be converted to ketones—the end-products of alcohol metabolism that make your morning-after breath raunchy, yet fruity.

Your body doesn't particularly enjoy breaking down acetone and acetate. The process disrupts your metabolism, causing such problems as blood sugar imbalances, abnormal electrolyte levels, and acid/base disturbances in your bloodstream. These, in turn, make you feel drunk, dehydrated, and ill.

Food slows down the absorption of alcohol, but antihistamines inhibit the enzyme alcohol dehydrogenase, so some allergy medications and OTC sleep aids might get you drunk faster than usual.

Once the alcohol passes through the gastrointestinal tract into the bloodstream, it enters the liver, where more alcohol dehydrogenase waits. Just as in the stomach cells, some of the alcohol is processed, and some continues into the rest of the body until it comes back full circle for another pass through the liver.

About 10 percent of what you drink never makes it all the way to acetone. Instead, it leaves the body via urine and exhaled air; hence the alcohol breath test. No matter how much you drink, the proportion of alcohol in the breath is directly related to the alcohol in the bloodstream. There's no way around it; this is one test you just can't beat.

Beyond the alcohol dehydrogenase pathway lies a backup system for metabolizing alcohol. This is called the microsomal ethanol oxidizing system (MEOS). In nondrinkers, this backup system doesn't play a big role in body functions, but the more you drink, the more your body builds up this system in response. What we call "tolerance" in people who have more than a couple of drinks a day is actually the metabolizing boost provided by this backup pathway.

WHAT HAPPENS WHEN YOU DRINK

Everyone's body differs, but here's what happens when the drinks start piling up.

Drinks per hour	You feel	Symptoms
<1 drink per hour	Fine	Nothing anyone else can see
1–2 drinks per hour	Happy	Euphoria or giddiness
		Increased sociability
		Loss of inhibitions
>2 drinks per hour	Sloppy	Poor memory and comprehension
		Slurred speech
		Clumsiness
3–4 drinks per hour	Loaded	Drowsiness
		Disorientation
		Nausea and vomiting
		Exaggerated emotions ("I love you!")
>4 drinks per hour	Trashed	Stupor
		Vomiting
		Incontinence

Drunk first aid for five, six, seven, or more drinks per hour: Call an ambulance if the person passes out. Make sure he's not lying on his back—one of the biggest preventable health problems a drunk faces is vomiting while intoxicated and the choking on the vomit. Keep the drunk warm, and don't let him wander off by himself if he's mobile. **Do not let this person, or anyone who has been drinking, near his or her car.**

Dealing with the Hangover

The bachelorette party was great, at least the parts you remember before you threw up in the taxi coming home. Now it's eight A.M., and after you've hauled yourself up off the bathroom floor where you were sleeping, you peer into your medicine chest, wondering what will ease the throbbing in your temples. You pick up a bottle of Tylenol and read the label to see how much to take. Lo and behold, the label warns you not to take the drug if you have more than three drinks a day. You certainly had more than three drinks last night. What gives?

Tylenol and Alcohol

Much has been made of the association between alcohol, Tylenol, and liver damage. Acetaminophen, the active ingredient in Tylenol and many other over-the-counter painkillers and cold remedies, is metabolized by the liver using some of the same enzymes that break down alcohol. When these enzymes are saturated, an accessory pathway breaks down the Tylenol; however, this secondary process leaves behind a metabolite that is toxic to the liver. At doses higher than 4 grams per day (eight extra-strength Tylenol) this pathway is activated and you raise your risk of toxic effects. Take too much Tylenol–10 grams, say, about a whole bottle–and you're quite likely to suffer liver damage. At 25 grams, you destroy your liver overnight.

I used to work in the liver transplant ward at the Scripps Clinic, and saw too many young people who didn't understand the science at play. They'd take a whole bottle of Tylenol to commit suicide. It's the easiest drug for a troubled young person to find, and these would-be suicide victims figured that taking a whole bottle of it must be deadly.

Unfortunately, you don't die. You destroy your liver, and end up spending weeks hanging on in the ICU in critical condition waiting for a liver transplant. Rather than a quick and painless exit from whatever caused the desire to die, these young people made their situations ten times worse.

While you can destroy your liver on a whole bottle of Tylenol, you won't cause liver damage on anything close to what a rational person might take for a headache–unless you are drinking.

Binge drinking can lower the toxic dose of Tylenol to as little as 4 grams in a day–eight pills–exactly what the maximum dose is on the bottle. At lower doses than the 4 grams, however, there have been no reports of liver failure associated with alcohol intake. So if you keep track of the number of Tylenol you're taking, you can in fact take Tylenol for a hangover.

Aspirin and Other Anti-inflammatories with Alcohol

Nonsteroidal anti-inflammatory drugs (NSAIDs) such as aspirin, ibuprofen, or naproxen to name a few, also have unintended effects on the body when combined with alcohol. Anti-inflammatories work by, as the name suggests, reducing inflammation. Take a sprained ankle. The ankle swells up and becomes warm as the body reacts to the stress and starts to heal. NSAIDs curb these reactions to stress, allowing the body to heal without the negative effects. NSAIDs are great painkillers, and even in the absence of inflammation can be wonderful for headaches.

There are just two potential downsides to anti-inflammatories for most people: Long-term use can cause kidney problems, and short- or longer-term use can cause stomach upset or ulcers. NSAID-related kidney problems are rare and associated with chronic use, such as for arthritis.

It's the ulcer issue that frightens most people. Over-the-counter anti-inflammatories inhibit an enzyme that maintains the protective lining of the stomach. Chronic use of these medications can cause that mucous lining to break down, allowing stomach acid to reach the surface. Alcohol also weakens the stomach's protective layer, so people who take a lot of NSAIDs and drink a lot increase their risk for bleeding stomach ulcers.

Given how unappetizing a bleeding stomach ulcer sounds, people try to reduce their risk by taking a "safe" NSAID such as aspirin. This is a misconception; aspirin is actually less safe than most other anti-inflammatories when it comes to ulcers. It's also usually less potent, so there are a couple of other medications you can find over the counter that can curb your headache and mitigate the risk of a bleeding ulcer.

One relatively safe nonprescription painkiller is ibuprofen (the generic drug sold under the names Advil and Motrin). You run the least risk of side effects (ulcers or liver damage) when you separate the alcohol from the drug by as much time as possible. So don't pop the pills before bed, but rather an hour or so before you need to be functioning in the morning.

For most healthy people without active ulcers or other medical problems, the maximum dose of ibuprofen is 800 mg, or four over-the-counter adult pills, three times a day. Companies tell you the maximum dose is two pills, to be on the safe side. The risk of damage from long-term use is much lower at this lower dose, but you aren't popping ibuprofen every day. You're popping it *today*, when your head is throbbing like you've got a polka band practicing in your cranium. Two pills are much less effective than four pills. The difference is like night and day. Double the dose, drink a ton of water, and you'll feel, if not like a million dollars, then at least like $75.

You can also take naproxen (Aleve) instead of aspirin.

If you are drinking regularly, or find yourself taking anti-inflammatories on a regular basis, it is a good idea to think about taking an over-the-counter medication to lower your risk of ulcers or gastritis (inflammation of the stomach lining). Prilosec (omeprazole) comes in a 20 mg dose over the counter. One or two pills a day blocks the acid in the stomach, lowering the risk of stomach problems dramatically. There aren't any real side effects, and you'll still be able to digest your food normally.

Doctor's note: If you have a history of ulcers or gastritis, or have severe abdominal pain, you should not only avoid all anti-inflammatories but avoid alcohol as well. While most anti-inflammatory use won't lead to ulcers (millions of people take them daily without problems), many bleeding ulcers are caused by anti-inflammatories. If you are at risk, or have any abdominal pain at all, it is better to be safe than sorry. See your doctor to find out for sure what you have.

Stopping a Hangover Before It Starts

You can take ibuprofen to ease your pain, but why wait until the next morning to fight a hangover? An ounce of prevention is worth at least a few ounces of cure. Follow these tips, and you'll be functional after a night of drinking a few hours earlier than you would be otherwise.

Before You Go Out

Make sure you are well-hydrated. Pre-party with a glass or two of something nonalcoholic. If you haven't been starving yourself, your kidneys should be maintaining a pretty efficient fluid balance, so a glass or two is all you need.

Have some food. Anything with calories is good, but the heavier the better. Go for the cheeseburger or fried mozzarella sticks—carbs and fats stay in the stomach longer than lean protein, giving them more time to absorb the alcohol when you drink. If you don't eat, you also run the risk of having low blood sugar in the morning after a long night metabolizing all the alcohol. Mind you, this method of mitigating hangover symptoms is not effective for weight loss.

While Drinking

Pace yourself. Your body metabolizes one drink an hour. Alternate a nonalcoholic beverage every other round, especially as the night heads toward a close.

Avoid caffeine while drinking, including cola drinks and energy drinks like Red Bull. Alcohol can keep you awake at night as it is; adding caffeine to the mix will only make you more dehydrated and less likely to sleep well.

Maintain your blood sugar by mixing your alcohol with some calories and sugar. Having a screwdriver instead of that diet vodka tonic will give your body more fuel to metabolize the alcohol. You can jog a little farther to burn the orange juice, and the heavy meal I just told you to have, later.

Stick to clear alcohols like vodka or gin. The alcohol fermentation process produces ethanol–the stuff that gets you drunk–and other metabolites such as acetaldehyde, methanol, propanol, and butanol. These metabolites, or "congeners," are found in higher concentrations in darker drinks such as bourbon, and in lower concentrations in clear alcoholic beverages such as vodka and gin.

While most of your hangover pain is due to alcohol, many of these congeners have an inflammatory effect on the body. Inflammation is associated with tissue damage and may account for some of the common symptoms of hangovers, such as nausea, weakness, tremors, diarrhea, headaches, and dry mouth. Fewer congeners should mean fewer symptoms . . . in theory. Drink too much, though, and you'll feel bad, whether your drink was dark as ink or clear as a windowpane.

After You Get Home

You may be craving pizza right now, so go ahead and have some food. You need complex carbs to slow the absorption of any alcohol still kicking around, and so you won't wake up starving the next morning.

Drink fluids such as Gatorade. You'll need to replace the electrolytes–like potassium and magnesium–that were depleted by your drinking. These small molecules are the chemical messengers of the body, and when the levels in your body are out of whack, everything else starts to malfunction.

Set your alarm to take 800 mg of ibuprofen or a couple of extra-strength Tylenol an hour or so before you need to be functional. Put a big glass of water by your bed and lay the pills by your alarm clock. You'll feel awful when you wake up to take them, but you'll feel much better an hour later.

Take some vitamins–a multivitamin with folic acid and B complex is essential to preserving good health when drinking. Most of the non-liver-related problems alcohol causes can be blamed on deficiencies in these vitamins.

Use a nasal spray. Sinus congestion interferes with your sleep patterns, and contributes to the headache and fatigue hangover victims feel in the morning. Afrin is a good choice for occasional use, since it works well and has no systemic side effects. If you use it daily, you can become dependent, but not if you use the spray just on occasion. Don't take an oral decongestant. These medications are stimulants and will interfere with your sleep, which is the last thing you want.

If you haven't had more than a few drinks, turn to the section on sleep in chapter 1, "Pushing the Limits," for a few tips on how to improve sleep after drinking. Although Ambien, Lunesta, and Sonata aren't approved for use with alcohol, when my patients ask, I tell them that these drugs are safe after a drink or two. If you've had more than that, or have any medical problems, speak with the doctor who prescribed the drug before you take it.

In the Morning

You should have short-circuited that splitting headache if you followed the advice above, but here are a few more tips:

Try not to chug coffee all day long. A cup in the morning will get you going and quell any caffeine-withdrawal headaches. More than a cup, though, will make your dehydration worse and add to your alcohol-withdrawal jitteriness. Trust me, that third or fourth cup is going to do more harm than good.

If your stomach is uneasy, you can take an over-the-counter antacid like Maalox or Tums. But if you have sharp stomach pain, call your doctor and have it checked out to make sure you don't have an ulcer or other serious damage.

Beware the "hair of the dog" cure. Drinking to cure a hangover does work like a charm, but it's tough to advocate it with a straight face. After a night of drinking, you're suffering, in part, from alcohol withdrawal. One more drink tapers you down slowly, and pushes some of the symptoms to later in the day. While treating the occasional Sunday hangover with a mimosa or bloody Mary at brunch doesn't hurt, if you need a shot of whiskey to get going every morning, you'd better get help.

Don't waste your time hunting for the perfect hangover pill.

There's only one herbal supplement that's been proven to help fight symptoms: extract of prickly pear cactus. A dose of 1,600 IU taken five hours before drinking has been shown to lower the number of hangover symptoms people had the next day. This supplement is sold on the Internet; just visit a vitamin site you like and you'll find plenty.

If you're ever bored in a library, studies on herbal supplements for hangovers are quite amusing to read. Researchers struggle to describe, in academic prose, the fact that they took a bunch of frat boys into a room with an open bar, gave them time to use it, then herded them all up at six A.M. to see whether they were functional. I did some stupid things to earn money in college, but I wish someone had paid me to participate in a study like this.

For the prickly pear cactus extract study, researchers rounded up a group of healthy adults and gave half of them the extract five hours before drinking, and a placebo to the other half. They then asked them to fill out a questionnaire the next day about symptoms, such as nausea and irritability. Two weeks later, the groups switched and did it again.

The end result was that the extract group did better on some, but not all, of the measures of hangover symptoms. The researchers also measured some markers of inflammation in the body, and found that the extract lowered such markers and that these markers were associated with reduced hangover symptoms.

This doesn't mean cactus extract is a cure-all. The study group had only slight improvements in symptoms, and they weren't allowed other treatments such as Advil or Tylenol during the study. But since the extract is safe, if not cheap, it's a low-risk way to reach for that holy grail of a hangover-free morning.

As for other commonly sold "hangover cures," I've heard it all. Unfortunately, despite the nearly $150 billion lost in wages to hangovers every year, the medical research on the subject is scant. Perhaps this is because no one, medical researchers included, has any incentive to fix a problem for which the cure is a day in front of the television or in bed.

In fact, the scant research on this topic is generally negative. The last decent hangover cure article I read was on artichoke extract. It was an excellent article. Unfortunately, it only proved that the stuff just doesn't work.

Other commonly touted cures are cysteine, "activated" calcium carbonate, vegetable carbon, and activated carbon. Of these substances, activated carbon is the most intriguing, because it's used in emergency rooms to treat people who have accidentally ingested toxins. The carbon molecules latch onto toxic substances in the stomach and intestines, preventing them from being absorbed, and helping them pass right through you. Unfortunately, activated carbon doesn't seem to work on alcohol, so hospitals don't use it in acute alcohol poisoning situations. If it doesn't work in hospitals, it's unlikely that the tiny amounts of activated carbon in hangover cure pills will work either.

The sad truth is that only time will sober you up. Even if you wind up in the hospital because you've passed out drunk, all the ER folks will do is watch you to make sure you don't choke on your vomit. Same thing with EMTs. Once when I was riding with the Hoboken Volunteer Ambulance Corps, we arrived on the scene of a motor vehicle accident outside the Lincoln Tunnel. The driver in question was so smashed that he tried to enter the Lincoln Tunnel going in the wrong direction and slammed head-on into a bus. Apparently he hadn't felt the crash. Though half his face was still embedded in the windshield, he was wandering around the street by the time we arrived.

If we didn't give this guy any medication for his alcohol intake, it's likely you won't need any either. A hangover is nature's way of teaching you, the hard way, to steer clear of alcohol poisoning and accidents. There is no magic pill to stop your pain.

Diagnosing a Drinking Problem

So far we've focused on casual drinkers and not on people with true drinking issues. Going out once or twice a week rarely leads to problems, but where do we draw the line? The answer varies, but a few warning signs indicate trouble. Psychologists call these the CAGE questions:

- Have you ever felt that you should CUT down on your drinking?
- Do you feel ANNOYED when people make comments to you about your drinking?
- Do you feel GUILTY about your drinking?
- Do you ever need an EYE-opener (a drink in the morning to get going again)?

Answering yes to any one of these questions spells trouble, but the more yes answers, the worse the problem. If the CAGE questions describe your drinking, then you should schedule an appointment with your doctor to talk about where this is heading–before someone else schedules the appointment for you.

Other signs that your drinking has become a problem include:

- Worrying about having enough alcohol to last through the night.
- Hiding alcohol or buying it at different stores so no one will know how much you are drinking.
- Sneaking drinks when others aren't looking.
- Blowing off responsibilities at work or at home because of drinking.
- Forgetting what happened while you were drinking.
- Not being able to stop drinking once you start.
- Hurting someone else as a result of your drinking.

Virtually everyone has experienced one or more of these signs at some point, usually at a college party gone crazy. The problem is when binge drinking becomes the norm. If you're getting falling down drunk more than a few times a year, it's time to assess the impact you're having on your health.

A SPECIAL MESSAGE TO FEMALE READERS:
YOUR SAFETY WHILE DRINKING

A few recent studies out of the University of Michigan and Penn State University show that young women's binge drinking rates now rival those of men. While I'm all for equality, I doubt this is what the suffragettes had in mind. Some women I know could drink me under the table, but in general, women will get drunker faster and suffer health effects at fewer drinks than men.

Drunk women also tend to attract drunk guys, and drunk guys don't have drunk women's best interests in mind. Crime rates rise and fall, but date rape is a constant problem. There's little worse than waking up Sunday morning in someone's bed and not knowing what you did with him, or knowing, but also knowing you were too drunk to stop it.

Make sure this doesn't happen to you by drinking on the buddy system. Go out with friends and make sure someone stays sober or is getting less drunk than the rest of you. Look out for one another. If you're pretty sure your friend wouldn't go home with a certain guy when she's sober, don't let her do it when she's drunk.

Don't be afraid to say "Stop it!" if someone's doing something you don't like. Don't worry about the niceties; chances are he's too drunk to remember if you offended him anyway. Leave parties in a group, not by yourself, and make sure you always have a safe way home. Keep cab fare and the number for a taxi service in your purse. Ask for help from a bouncer or bartender if you need it. And if you feel yourself getting close to the drunken edge, back up, stop drinking, eat something, and switch to water. There will be more parties. Better to lose your buzz than have this be the party you spend years trying to forget.

Drinking, Smoking, Staying Healthy

Life is often stressful. Everyday vices such as smoking and drinking can make life more manageable. Dealing with stressful situations head-on is better in the long run, but I, too, have smoked. I drink. I won't begrudge anyone a few moments with these vices. The key is keeping it all in check.

Moderation is often a virtue, but with everyday vices such as drinking and smoking, moderation is practically a religion unto itself. A few drinks a week are good for you. A few cigarettes won't necessarily land you in the cancer ward if you practice moderation and quit on time. The key is making sure you don't smoke long enough or drink enough that these vices add to your stress levels themselves. Smoking and drinking are supposed to be pleasurable. If they're leading to risky sex, wicked hangovers, falling down the stairs, or sucking wind when you try to run a mile, then they're not so pleasurable. In that case, it's time to talk to your doctor or a substance abuse counselor on ways you can cut back—or quit.

Three

Dieting: Keeping Safe While Slimming Down

EVERY DOCTOR'S got a diet these days. Bookshelves in the diet section have been gaining weight with the rest of America, so if you want a branded plan (South Beach, Weight Watchers, Ornish) you have plenty of choices. I'm not going to load you down with recipes and menus. If the only ingredients in your refrigerator are a bottle of soy sauce and leftovers of last night's take-out Chinese, a recipe for garlic-seared flank steak with pesto-stuffed tomatoes will inspire nothing but the desire to grab a bag of chips.

Instead, this chapter looks at the basics of a healthy diet and exercise plan that will help you trim down over time. Then we'll look at how to lose *a bit* of weight quickly on an eight-week crash diet.

The bad news is that changing your weight for life involves changing your life for good. The good news is that if you want to drop ten pounds in a few weeks for a wedding or beach vacation, you can do so without damaging your health, as long as you don't mind that you'll probably regain most of the weight by the time you get your photos back.

Losing It for Good

You can't open a newspaper these days without reading about America's weight problem. You can't go to a mall without seeing it firsthand. Even in New York City, home of the slim and glamorous, I've seen many patients who have packed on the pounds over the years through sedentary desk jobs, lack of exercise, excessive drinking, and poor eating habits. The unfortunate ones suffer from blood sugar imbalances and then, as things get worse, diabetes. Over time, excess pounds can lead to heart disease, fatigue, joint pain, and other problems.

No one likes being fat. But few people want to hear that losing large amounts of weight–thirty pounds or more–involves changing *everything* about their life. You have to learn to let go of comfort foods, learn ways to manage stress other than eating, understand that portion size counts, and learn how to exercise, even if you've grown stiff and awkward from years of inactivity.

Even some of my diabetic patients, for whom weight loss is more about health than vanity, look for that magic pill that will change their size. One diabetic man I've treated was admitted to the hospital twice in a year with soaring blood glucose levels. Shortly after his second discharge, he came to see me. When we got around to discussing diet, he told me that his breakfast consisted of lemon meringue pie that was left over from the night before. He was sheepish, but he insisted it was a special occasion. It turns out, however, that each week brought a special occasion, from dinner with clients to a cousin's visit to his sister's birthday.

Some people even prefer the scalpel to the grueling process of burning off excess weight; witness the popularity of gastric bypass surgery. One in two hundred patients (or more, depending on the study) dies within a month of surgery, yet many overweight people still choose this option, hoping that surgically altering their stomachs and guts will take the hard decisions about changing their lives out of their hands.

But as people with newly stapled stomachs discover, losing weight is still hard work. It's hard work if you're seriously overweight, and it's hard work even if you're not.

My first experience with serious weight loss came in a very different guise than the chronic obesity cases I see now. One of my friends in medical school, Paul, was into bodybuilding, and he decided, some time in our second year, that it was time to push his body into competitive form.

Mind you, Paul wasn't fat. Before his first contest, he clocked in at 9 percent body fat, which is excellent for a guy. Fit women average about 21 to 24 percent body fat, and fit men 14 to 17 percent. To be a serious competitor, though, Paul had to reach his target of 4 percent body fat. For that, he had to make some serious lifestyle changes. Since your cells are surrounded by lipids, which are fats, 4 percent is about as low as you can go and stay aboveground.

My friend didn't want to lose any lean muscle mass, just fat. Diets can make you lose both, but there are some ways to adjust your diet to give the body as much protein as possible while removing enough calories to cause the body to burn its fat stores.

So, way before low-carbohydrate diets were mainstream, Paul cut his simple carb count down to just a few grams a day–no white breads, pasta, potatoes, or packaged snack foods. Fat was banned. He grilled all his meats or pan cooked them using fat-free cooking spray. He steamed or boiled his vegetables. He ate a bit of brown rice and other fiber-rich grains but cut out sugars completely. It is amazing how few calories lean meats, vegetables, and other fiber-rich foods contain. You can eat sensible meals, and a few snacks, and still take in only 1,000 to 1,500 calories a day. With this low a caloric intake, and with his two-hour lifting sessions, Paul's veins were showing through his skin in no time.

As he discovered, the foods that have made up the human diet since our hunter-gatherer days are healthy. It's just what we do to make the roughage palatable that ruins the healthy part. Sauces, toppings, and processing all add sugars and fats, which add up to more calories. More calories minus more exercise equals a physique that's less like a hunter-gatherer's and more like those of the woolly mammoths our ancestors were hunting.

The key to losing weight is burning more calories than you take in. Anyone who tells you that you can eat like a horse and still tip the scale in a negative direction is pulling your leg. That goes for diets that involve eating bacon, pork chops, and egg yolks, or those that tell you to feast on rice cakes and fat-free cookies.

The average person burns between 1500 and 2500 calories a day just being alive. Exercise ups this number a bit. But the bounty of American supermarkets and restaurants conspires to help you shovel far more than 1,500 to 2,500 calories a day into your mouth. A double cheeseburger with fries and a twelve-ounce Coke set you back more than 1,000 calories. Two beers after work plops on another 500 calories. Even a "coffee"–say, a Starbucks mocha malt frappuccino with whipped cream–can pack nearly 600 calories. Eat a slice of cake with that coffee drink and you may as well have ordered fried Twinkies with a side of lard.

Most of us aren't even remotely aware of how many calories we're taking in, and so it's no wonder that our weight creeps up year after year. We're lucky we aren't porking up faster when you calculate the average American's daily caloric expenditure from exercise. How far do you walk from your car to your desk? Is the remote one foot away from your spot on the couch or two?

The first step to permanent weight loss is to make an honest accounting of your current diet. Buy a calorie-counting book and carry it everywhere for a few days, recording everything you eat *and drink* along with the number of calories. Prepared foods give you this number on the Nutrition Facts label. Just make sure you're measuring your serving sizes accurately. If that bag of chips says it contains 2.5 servings, and you eat the whole bag, do the math. For foods you don't know–such as an order of take-out kung-pao chicken–estimate based on the likely ingredients. You may not know what's in the sauce, but you can see whether the chicken is fried and how much rice you're inhaling. Several Web sites, such as CaloriesCount.org, or NutritionData.com, list the calorie counts for thousands of foods, including those on popular restaurant menus.

Keeping this tally will uncover weak spots you may not have thought about. A mindless pass by the pantry can result in your eating a 300-calorie handful of Doritos that never registers in your conscious count for the day.

Once you know exactly what you're eating, you can eliminate the empty calories, which I define as calories from simple sugars, starches, or fats that lack enough benefits (in the form of fiber, vitamins, proteins, or minerals) to justify the hit. Try these simple changes:

Eliminate simple sugars. Simple sugars are absorbed by the body so quickly that they cause your blood sugar levels to spike. The spike is followed, an hour or two later, by a crash as your pancreas reacts to the increase in blood sugar by secreting insulin into the bloodstream. The insulin clears the blood sugar by turning it into storage forms: glycogen for short-term storage in muscles, and fat for the long term. Not only does this fat add to what you've got to lose, but the insulin invariably drops blood sugar so fast that you end up having *too little*. This crash makes you feel ravenous and more likely to grab the first edible object you see. Better to avoid foods made of simple sugars as much as possible. Sodas and juices, for instance, have too much sugar and too little nutritional value to justify keeping them in your diet; replace them with water or diet beverages. Even such healthy-sounding drinks as "vitamin water" can be full of sugar, so make no assumptions. Candy and desserts can be eliminated or pared back to just a bite to satisfy a craving.

You also need to watch out for foods with hidden sugars. Check the label: Is high-fructose corn syrup listed as an ingredient? If so, the food has little chance of being good for you. Satisfy your sweet tooth with whole fruits such as strawberries, apples, pears, or pineapples. While fruits do have sugar, they also contain fiber, which slows sugar's absorption.

Pare back starches. Like sugar, starches such as white bread, white rice, pasta, and potatoes are absorbed rapidly and cause insulin levels to spike. You don't have to eliminate these foods completely, but you should limit your consumption to one small portion a day.

Watch the fat. Fats store energy in the body. They pack twice as many calories per gram as other foods, thus giving your body ample reserves to make it through the lean times. Yet with a McDonald's on every corner, a famine doesn't appear to be imminent for most Americans, so saturated fats (think butter and other fats that are solid at room temperature) and transfats (margarine) are an easy source of calories to cut. Since you do need *some* fat–for taste, texture, and survival–try substituting healthier monounsaturated fats, such as olive oil and canola oil, for the butter and bacon grease you may have been eating. People who eat diets rich in monounsaturated fats have a lower incidence of heart disease and stroke than those whose diets tilt toward the saturated side.

Below is a list of the different kinds of fats with examples of foods that contain each. The first two fats are pretty healthy; the last two are not. That said, fat is fat, and even good fats pack just as many calories as the bad ones.

Omega-3 fatty acid	fatty fish (salmon, trout, sardines, albacore tuna, herring), tofu or soybeans, canola oil, flaxseed oil, walnuts
Monounsaturated or polyunsaturated fats	olive, canola, or peanut oil, avocados, safflower, sesame, soy, corn, or sunflower oils
Transfats	partially hydrogenated vegetable oils (most processed foods, such as cookies, crackers, cakes, and french fries)
Saturated fats	whole milk, cream, cheese, butter, palm oil, coconut oil, or cocoa butter

Avoid alcohol. I know this is tough if you want a social life while dieting. Just keep in mind that a beer on tap packs over 200 calories, a *small* margarita or piña colada can top 300, and *any* alcohol will lower your metabolism–exactly what you don't need when you are trying to lose weight. So stick to one or two drinks a day at most, and unless you're drinking all night and need the sugar, go for lower-calorie drinks. A shot of hard liquor has about 40 calories. Wine is also a good choice, or mixed drinks with diet sodas. If you must have beer, go for light or ultra-light varieties.

What to Eat

Your diet should now consist mostly of the following:

Complex Carbohydrates

Thanks to the South Beach diet craze, such phrases as "good carbs" and "bad carbs" have entered everyday conversation. If simple sugars (think doughnuts, white rice, chocolate cake with fudge frosting) are the bad carbs, complex carbohydrates (think whole oats, brown rice, and whole-grain breads) are the good carbs. These foods' complex molecular structures take longer to break down than sugar, so they are absorbed more slowly in the intestinal tract and do not cause the same blood sugar spike that simple sugars cause.

In general, you can distinguish between good and bad carbs by looking at the food's color. White carbs have been processed to remove the fiber. Brown carbs have the roughage intact. While this rule isn't perfect—brown-colored table sugar is still just sugar—it does help.

Complex carbohydrates are an excellent source of energy and nutrients. You still can't eat all you'd like if you want to lose weight, but if your weight is stable, you can enjoy your whole-wheat pasta and no-sugar-added granola guilt free.

Fiber

Vegetables and fruits are essential to weight loss and healthy weight maintenance. For starters, vegetables and fruits are packed with vitamins and minerals. But more important for weight loss, these foods have tons of fiber, which keeps the intestinal tract regular and provides a feeling of fullness with far fewer calories than sugar or fat. Every meal should include these foods. Just don't drench your asparagus in butter or you're missing the point. Currently, the USDA recommends four and a half cups of fruits and vegetables per day on a 2,000-calorie diet. It's tough to overdo it when it comes to fiber.

Protein

Protein is the building block of the human body. It builds and maintains muscle, aids in digestion, helps ward off infection, and (as part of the body's enzymes) helps you respond to stimuli. Certain amino acids derived from protein also give a feeling of satiety, or fullness. This is why a bag of peanut M&M's fills you up faster than the plain ones.

Meats, fish, poultry, and tofu are all good sources of protein. The trick is to keep the fat content low at the same time. Seafood and white meats tend to have lower fat contents than red meats (including pork). Oily fish such as salmon and red snapper also contain heart-friendly omega-3 fatty acids.

You should eat some protein with every meal, and every snack if you can. Unfortunately, cooking up a small slice of red snapper for that midmorning coffee break isn't usually an option.

To fill the gap, many health food stores sell protein-based supplements such as shakes, powders, and bars. I'm a fan of the low-calorie versions—I make myself a protein shake for an afternoon snack most days—but be sure to read the label. Some 250-calorie high-protein bars have only 9 or so grams of protein. At just 4 calories per gram of protein, that means you've got 200 plus calories from sugars and fats sneaking in with your supposedly healthy snack. Aim for 100 to 150 calories per snack, and make sure your protein supplement has at least one gram of protein for every 10 calories.

Making Healthy Choices

By sticking with lean proteins, complex carbs, and fruits and vegetables, you're unlikely to accumulate enough calories in a day to gain weight. If you're exercising as well, you will gradually lose weight.

This sounds simple, but it isn't easy. Sweets and fats taste good. Grilling meats and vegetables takes more time than grabbing a bucket of fried chicken or a cheesy burrito on the way home from work. Sometimes, tough schedules and long commutes mean you get so desperately hungry that you inhale a cheeseburger, pizza, or whatever is nearby. You can eat healthfully and lose weight despite a hectic, on-the-go life, but you do need to think about when and what you're going to eat before the situation becomes desperate.

Snacking is key. People snack for all sorts of reasons—when they're hungry, out of habit while watching TV, when they're nervous, or for emotional solace. You can't control all the triggers that make you want to stick your hand in the Cheez-Its box. But you can minimize the likelihood that you'll munch on things you shouldn't.

For starters, don't keep your trigger foods in the house. I'm not saying you'll never eat ice cream again. I'm saying that if you have a habit of eating the whole container of Häagen-Dazs when it's in the fridge, force yourself to go to a convenience store to buy a small serving when you have a craving. You'll likely decide it isn't worth the effort.

Second, fill your fridge or pantry with healthy snacks. Precut fruits and vegetables are more expensive than their whole counterparts in the produce aisle, but you're also more likely to eat them. So think of it as an investment in your body. Nuts in moderation are good; parcel them into individual-serving-size bags (1 ounce) so you won't keep your hand in the cashew jar. Meal replacement shakes and bars are quick and easy if you've got a taste for them. Just check the label to be sure you're not eating a cleverly disguised candy bar by accident.

Most important, don't skip meals, and don't wait until you're starving to eat or you'll lack all sense of control. Here are some meal and snack suggestions to get you going. The only special equipment you'll need is a set of measuring cups. Portion size *does* matter. Every serving should fit in a one-cup measure. Breakfasts and snacks can be, total, one to two servings. Lunch and dinner can have two to four servings.

BREAKFAST

- 1 cup whole-grain cereal such as Total, or soy-rich cereal such as Kashi, with skim milk and up to one cup of fruit
- Oatmeal topped with a bit of cinnamon and granola for crunch, and fruit
- Scrambled egg whites with whole-wheat toast and turkey breast or lean ham
- Egg-white omelette with low-fat cheese and chopped vegetables
- Low-fat, artificially sweetened yogurt with fruit and low-sugar granola or Grape-Nuts or other high-fiber cereal

• Have coffee with skim milk and Splenda or other artificial sweetener with any of the above

LUNCH

• 3 to 4 ounces (a quarter pound) of turkey, chicken breast, or tuna fish on whole-grain bread with lettuce and tomato and fruit
• Vegetable, bean, or chicken soup with fruit and toast
• Salad bar: dark greens, grilled chicken, tuna, or turkey; a bit of cheese and as many veggies as you can load on. Skip the croutons and substitute a few nuts for crunch. Put the dressing on the side and dip your fork in it before spearing the lettuce.
• Soy burger or turkey burger with a piece of fruit or side of veggies
• Have diet soda or tea, Crystal Light, or water (tap or mineral) with any of the above

SNACKS

• Precut pineapple, strawberries, melon, grapes, oranges, blueberries, or any other fruit
• Apple or celery with peanut butter
• 1 ounce (a small handful) of almonds, cashews, peanuts, or walnuts
• Carrots or celery with low-fat ranch dip or hummus
• Sliced turkey with cheese
• Low-fat cottage cheese on whole-grain crackers
• Protein bar or protein shake (low-fat yogurt, fruit, and protein powder)

DINNER

Eating out? There are healthy options everywhere.

DELI

• Sliced turkey or grilled chicken sandwich on whole-grain bread with side of fruit or veggies
• Grilled chicken on a salad with veggies, nuts, and a vinegar-and-olive-oil dressing
• Chicken, bean, or vegetable soup with either of these options

Chinese restaurant

- Steamed chicken with broccoli, brown rice (one cup or less), and soy sauce
- Pepper steak with mixed vegetables, brown rice, and sauce on the side

Japanese restaurant

- Miso soup and salad with one California, tuna, or salmon roll, or a few pieces of sashimi

Burger joint

- Grilled chicken sandwich with side salad
- Dinner-size salad with dressing on the side, add grilled chicken if possible
- Regular-size hamburger with lettuce, tomato, pickle, and mustard (no mayo)—remove half the bun to cut some starch calories or ask for it on wheat toast
- Veggie burger or turkey burger with lettuce, tomato, pickle, and mustard
- Diet cola or bottled water

Italian restaurant

- Minestrone soup and salad
- Grilled chicken parmesan—scrape off some of the cheese
- Any chicken or seafood dish with a red or clear sauce, and pasta (one cup)—avoid white or pink sauces, as they're usually made with cream

Greek/Mediterranean restaurant

- Grilled chicken, lamb, or beef kabobs, grilled vegetables, and brown rice (one cup)
- Avoid the gyro in favor of grilled meats and vegetables
- Any broiled or grilled fish

Mexican restaurant

- Bean or chicken burrito with brown rice and a side salad
- Small grilled chicken, beef, or fish taco loaded with lettuce

and tomato. Go easy on cheese and skip the sour cream in favor of a little guacamole. The avocado is tasty, filling, and good for your cholesterol.

INDIAN

• Tandoori chicken with rice and wheat naan bread, no butter.

AT HOME

Mix one serving of lean meat with two or three servings of vegetables/fruits or two vegetables/fruits plus one starch. Aim to make most of your dinners from fish or white meats. Try:

• 6 ounces baked, poached, or broiled fish of your choice, plus one cup cooked carrots plus a small salad, and a cup of melon for dessert
• 4 ounces London broil with green beans and a sweet potato plus strawberries for dessert
• 4 ounces tenderloin with asparagus, baked yam, and pineapple for dessert
• 1 cup whole-wheat spaghetti with ground turkey and tomato sauce loaded with peppers, onions, and mushrooms, plus salad
• Stir-fried chicken and vegetables with one cup brown rice plus fruit for dessert

Jazzing It Up

Condiments and spices add a lot of flavor for not a lot of calories. Horseradish, for example, perks up salmon faster than butter, and doesn't pack on the pounds. Ginger adds zest to chicken. Hot pepper, hot sauce, or salsa makes any food taste better. Lemon juice and balsamic vinegar marinate meat in a pinch. Olive oil and canola oil add healthy fats to a diet, so cook with these or with cooking spray. Cinnamon sweetens your food, as do sugar substitutes, for far fewer calories than sugar itself. Ketchup, teriyaki, and barbecue sauces tend to have a lot of sugar, so use these sparingly. Mustard is good. Mayonnaise loads on the fat.

A Few More Tips

Water is the best drink for you—it keeps you hydrated and it's calorie-free. If water gets boring, add a slice of lemon or lime for zest, or try sparkling water for fizz.

When in doubt, read the labels. Eat slowly, chewing every bite, and drink lots of water. You'll feel full faster. If you find yourself longing for something bad for you, chew a piece of sugar-free gum or have some sugar-free Jell-O and see if the urge passes. If not, you can have a bite, then throw the rest away. Yes, this is wasteful, but if you're worried about starving children in China, write a check to your favorite charity. Getting fat won't help these starving children at all.

A Note on Motivation

Like any diet, this eating plan is a bit austere. If you're serious about weight loss, though, you have to realize you can't do it without sacrifice. Be cynical anytime you see an ad featuring a smiling woman who lost weight "without trying" on some miracle plan. In every case, the success story busted her ass for months working out and cutting calories and then attributed her weight loss to whoever is paying the bills.

Exercise—and sometimes medication—is part of weight loss and maintenance. But unless you're getting a job as an aerobics instructor, it's tough to fit enough exercise into a day to make you lose weight without cutting calories, too.

Like quitting smoking, giving up bad eating habits takes a phenomenal amount of willpower. Every day you'll be tempted to cheat. So think about everything you put in your mouth. Eat one slice of cheese instead of two, whole-grain bread instead of white, a cup of rice instead of more. None of this is easy. But as my friend from medical school discovered when he achieved the physique he wanted, eating better has its obvious rewards. There's nothing like watching the weight come off to banish the Twinkies from your pantry and the soda from your fridge.

Exercise

Exercise is the second pillar of weight loss. The average person burns between 1,500 and 2,500 calories a day. This is called the basal metabolic rate (BMR). Men tend to have higher BMRs because muscle burns more calories than fat, and men have more muscle mass than women, but BMRs vary across ages and ethnicities. Everyone is different. The differences mean some people stay thin despite lousy eating habits, and some people struggle to beat back obesity their whole lives.

No matter what your BMR is, though, the good news is that this is not the final word on the matter. Exercising is the gift that keeps giving when it comes to your metabolism.

If you've ever hopped on a treadmill, you've seen the meter counting calories as you go. During a twenty-minute run, for instance, the average person burns about 250 calories. But your body doesn't stop working when your twenty minutes are done. Exercise actually raises your basal metabolic rate for the next twenty-four to forty-eight hours. This means you keep burning more calories than you would otherwise, long after you've showered and retired to the couch.

There are two types of exercise: cardiovascular (the kind that makes you out of breath), and muscle building. If you're trying to lose weight long term, you should do mostly cardio, with some light weight training thrown in. You want to stay away from the low-repetition, high-resistance weight lifting that builds muscle. There's nothing wrong with this kind of exercise, it's just that with weight loss, burning calories should be your first priority.

For now, stick to activities that involve constant movement for at least twenty to thirty minutes most days of the week, and make sure you break a sweat. You can run, walk, bike, swim, row, skip, whatever. To shake things up and keep your body balanced, you might want to mix in cardio activities that work your arms (swimming, rowing, elliptical trainers) with those that work your legs.

If you've got problem spots, don't bother doing endless repetitions of spot-toning exercises such as sit-ups. Your sleek, toned stomach won't show until you burn the two inches of fat on top of it.

Aside from that, the most important exercise tip is to just do it, and then keep pushing yourself to do it longer and harder every day.

If you're a newbie, start with a daily fifteen- to twenty-minute brisk walk. Even if it's just taking a walk around the parking lot during your lunch break, any little bit helps. If you haven't worked out in ages, or you feel any problems while exercising, see your doctor for a checkup before getting started. But I'm guessing she'll say the same thing I am: Just go for it.

People have a great deal of inertia; if you spend more than a few days away from the gym, you soon feel like you may as well not go back. So I advise my patients that if they don't feel like exercising, go to the gym anyway and stand there and hang out for ten minutes. *Half of success is showing up.* Try not to take more than a day off a week; if you can't go to the gym, go for a walk. You'll have good days and bad days, but the important thing is to build a habit where your day doesn't feel right if you haven't broken a sweat. If you're the kind of person who finds it easier to say yes to other people than to yourself, make a standing date to work out with your partner or a friend, so you're in the doghouse if you don't show.

It's amazing how addictive exercise can become. When you push yourself further–break a ten-minute mile for the first time, or swim half an hour without stopping–you feel on top of the world. You want more. *Give in to that temptation.* Soon you can start adding weight lifting to tone and build your muscles. Ask a buff friend to show you around the machines at the gym. Or buy a set of weights and some exercise tapes. Or use your body for resistance (push-ups and chin-ups build upper-body strength *quickly*).

Once you've established a regular exercise routine, start looking for other ways to incorporate exercise into your day. Walk around the halls at work. Take the stairs. Park in the back of the lot. Stretch at your desk. Anything that gets the blood pumping will lead to a leaner you.

Dietary Supplements

All diets involve changing or restricting what you eat. While plenty of people don't get enough vitamins and minerals in a normal diet, it's even tougher if you're cutting calories. So the one supplement that's essential to a diet is a daily multivitamin with thiamine, folate, iron, calcium, and magnesium.

When it comes to diet supplements, though, people generally aren't talking about vitamins. Given the number of people trying to lose weight without trying too hard, companies can make millions on herbal supplements that claim to help you on the path. Ephedra, for instance, had a heyday in drug and health food store sales, but enthusiasm waned when people had an alarming number of strokes and heart attacks after taking it.

After the FDA pulled ephedra from the market, the companies that had been hawking ephedra rushed to replace it with other "miracle" supplements. The active ingredients in all these supplements are derivatives of caffeine, a stimulant. While most of these supplements aren't more dangerous than a cup of coffee, they won't help your weight loss any more than coffee will, either.

The only supplements I've seen positive evidence for are chromium, fenugreek seeds, and soy protein. Chromium is a trace nutrient found in many natural food sources, including meats, fish, whole grains, cheese, and many vegetables. Chromium appears to increase insulin receptor sensitivity, and decrease insulin resistance. This means fewer spikes in blood sugar. This doesn't mean that chromium will cancel out a bowl of Cap'n Crunch. It means that chromium, with a low-sugar diet, may help you eat less than you might otherwise.

Fenugreek seeds and soy protein also affect blood sugar levels. Fenugreek seeds increase the body's ability to process glucose. Soy protein slows the absorption of glucose from the intestinal tract, in much the same way fiber does. The recommended doses are 1–2 grams of fenugreek seeds a day, usually in a capsule, and as much soy protein as you can manage in your diet.

Adding soy protein to your meals will take some work–the American diet just isn't that high in it. Soy-rich foods include tofu, miso soup, soybeans (edamame), soy milk, and the soy-protein powders sold in nutrition stores. You can find a wider variety of soy products at Asian grocery stores, if you live near one. The biggest downside to soy is that some people are intolerant and suffer abdominal cramping or gas. If this is you, just forget about it. You won't stick with a diet change that makes you miserable.

The important thing to keep in mind with these supplements is you won't see major changes. Diet and exercise are the cake, everything else is icing. Even my colleagues who run weight-loss centers don't recommend buying supplements. They just aren't that helpful. So pop a daily multivitamin, but beyond that, I don't recommend wasting your money.

Medications

Unlike herbal supplements, some prescription medications actually do make you lose weight rapidly. Some, such as Topamax for seizure disorders, have other indications but can be used for weight loss. Metformin, a drug diabetic patients take to lower their blood sugar, can also help you lose pounds. But in general, since these drugs have not been FDA approved for weight loss, and don't work any better than other medications that have been approved and studied for this purpose, it is usually a good move to start with one of the approved weight-loss agents unless your doctor suggests otherwise.

Many of the approved weight-loss agents are stimulants, which work by taking advantage of the body's fight-or-flight response. When adrenaline courses through your veins, your body responds by reducing appetite. If you're about to run for your life, after all, your body has no interest in chilling out and grabbing a burger. Stimulants cause the same response.

People generally feel a boost of energy after taking stimulants. These drugs can also increase your blood pressure, and make you feel jittery, or make you stay awake when you want to sleep. You can mitigate these side effects by starting with a low dose and working up gradually, and by taking the drugs first thing in the morning to avoid insomnia.

Phentermine and phendimetrazine are two typical drugs in this class. Other stimulants, such as Ritalin, do the trick as well. Phentermine is my favorite for patients without any health problems beyond their weight (it isn't recommended for those with heart arrhythmia or those on multiple antidepressants). This drug got a bad reputation when people used it as part of the famous Phen-fen weight-loss combo, but the negative side effects were caused by the "fen"–fenfluramine–not the "phen"–phentermine. With phentermine, you can double the rate at which you lose weight. On a strict diet and exercise program, the average person loses about 8 percent of his or her body weight in a year. With phentermine, this doubles to 15 percent (for a 200-pound person, this is about 30 pounds).

Other Drugs

A few other classes of drugs can help you lose weight, too. Meridia was originally marketed as an antidepressant, but it turned out to work better for weight loss than depression. This drug works by inhibiting the uptake of norepinephrine and serotonin, causing a decrease in appetite and an increase in satiety. This means you feel fuller and more satisfied after a meal. Meridia is often used for patients who are quite obese and need a long-term drug regimen, because it is generally safe and well tolerated.

Wellbutrin, another antidepressant, is often used for smoking cessation, but it curbs all sorts of cravings, including cravings for food.

The last medication to consider is Xenical, which works by blocking fat absorption in your gut. Eat 10 grams of fat while taking Xenical and you only absorb 7. The downside is that those 3 grams of fat have to go somewhere, namely, out the other end. If you eat a greasy cheeseburger with 30 grams of fat, the 9 that don't get absorbed grease up your intestines, sometimes to the point of fecal incontinence.

This is just as gross as it sounds. When I was working in California, one of the Xenical reps I met experienced this firsthand. He popped a pill and ate two slices of pizza before driving home on the infamous San Diego freeways. He got stuck in four lanes of bumper-to-bumper traffic and spent the next two hours doubled over in the driver's seat trying to maintain control of his sphincter. He finally had to toss his trousers when Xenical won the battle.

If you can stick to a low-fat diet, Xenical can speed your weight loss. Cheat, and you'll learn in an unpleasant way that you shouldn't have done that.

> **Doctor's note:** Given the multibillion-dollar diet market, it's no wonder that legitimate pharmacies aren't the only places hawking diet drugs such as phentermine, Meridia, and Xenical. You might have e-mail messages in your in-box right now offering to sell you these drugs. Don't go for it. For starters, it's illegal to sell or purchase these drugs without a prescription. Plus, you might be taking another drug that would interact with these, or you might have some other condition that would make stimulants or antidepressants problematic. But on top of that, these operations tend to be ridiculously expensive and not exactly concerned with quality control. You run a good chance of not getting what you ordered and being fleeced in the process.

The Eight-Week Crash Diet

When people first hear that there are a few drugs that can speed their weight loss, they have one of two reactions. Either they freak out because they can't handle the thought of interfering with their bodies this way, or they salivate at the prospect of doubling their progress.

My first caveat before telling you how to incorporate drugs into a crash diet is that drugs alone will not make you thin. I've got a recently divorced patient in her mid-forties, Wendy, who wanted to slim down before she entered the dating scene. She did her homework and came in looking for medications. She was an excellent candidate, and so I put her on phentermine with the caveat that she embark on a rigorous diet and exercise program. Wendy assured me she would follow my directions, but as soon as she left the office she decided to dispense with the diet and exercise and just go with the drugs. Four months later, she hadn't dropped a pound. After that, we pulled the plug on phentermine and she went looking for another miracle cure.

Medications without diet and exercise are basically useless. Multiple trials have proven this, and so I rarely recommend diet drugs to someone who hasn't demonstrated a willingness to ramp up the exercise and modify her plate.

How It Works

Crash dieting isn't an ideal way to lose weight. If you're not obese, it's tough to lose more than a pound a week from diet and exercise, so you need at least three months to drop ten pounds. Unfortunately, wedding invitations, vacation worries, and the realization of an impending college reunion all hit right around six to eight weeks before the event. That's when the person (I'll say "she" because it usually is) panics and decides to get serious.

I see a fair number of these would-be crashers in my office. The question is usually sheepish: "Is there a way I can lose ten to fifteen pounds before . . . my niece's bat mitzvah, my sister's wedding, my trip to Tahiti?"

My medical textbooks would tell me to break out the sensible diet advice from the first part of this chapter. But I believe medicine is, at least in part, about giving patients information and empowering them to make their own health choices. While in general it's wiser to lose weight slowly and in a way that can be sustained long term, I'm glad these dieters come to see me. Most people who attempt drastic diets are too embarrassed to seek medical help, and wind up buying dangerous supplements or drugs, or cutting so many calories they do real harm to themselves. If a woman is in my office, on the other hand, we have a good chance of achieving her goals without harming her health.

So here's what I did with one patient, Maria, when she came in to talk about weight loss. Expecting the standard slightly overweight desk-bound professional, I was surprised to walk into the room and meet one of the most glamorous women I have ever seen in real life. Maria, a Brazilian model, had come to America a few months earlier for a cover shoot, and had been working steadily ever since. The only problem was that she'd also discovered the American diet, and had put on a few pounds. While my inexpert eyes wouldn't have guessed she was too heavy to model, her agency had told her that her career rode on dropping fifteen pounds—yesterday.

On the one hand, I thought her agency was being silly. On the other, I also didn't want this ambitious young woman to lose her job, and hence be deported. So here's what we did:

- **Cut calories—drastically.** You need about 1,000 calories a day to survive. If you drop your intake below that, your body strains to maintain its blood sugar and electrolyte levels. You also run the risk of nutrient deficiencies. Low levels of potassium, sodium, magnesium, and other minerals lead to nerve and muscle problems that can be incapacitating or deadly. But you don't actually need much more than 1,000 calories a day, at least in the short term. Maria kept track of everything she ate and cut her intake to 1,200 calories a day, mainly soups—made with vegetables for bulk and beans, chicken, or fish for protein—and salads. She tried to maintain the right level of vitamins and minerals by using darker greens (spinach, for instance, instead of iceberg lettuce) and varying the colors of her veggies and fruits, but to be sure, she also took a multivitamin every day.

- **Upped the exercise—drastically.** To lose weight, you need to do at least twenty to thirty minutes of cardiovascular activity (such as running) most days of the week. There is no maximum amount of activity, so if you can go for an hour, you should. Maria would alternate running and walking for an hour a day, and do a half hour of weight training as well. With an exercise program like this, she was burning hundreds of extra calories a day.

Keep in mind that calories fuel the body. If you're cutting calories, you'll have less fuel—and a lot less energy. Don't be surprised if you have trouble exercising at first. As your body adjusts to the lower intake, you will have more energy and can increase the duration and intensity of your workouts. Plan your two biggest meals two hours before and an hour after you exercise to maximize your energy and your results.

To make the numbers come out right for weight loss, you need to burn 500 to 1,000 calories more per day than you take in. If your BMR is 1,500 calories a day and you're eating 1,000, you're good. If you bump your burn rate to 2,000 calories a day, you can lose about eight pounds a month—and that's before we get to the prescription medications that can augment your results.

- **Hydrated her system.** If you're trying to lose weight, you need to drink a lot of water. Not only does staying hydrated help your muscles and tissues maintain adequate blood flow, if you're working out and eating a lot of protein, your kidneys have to work harder, and they need water to function as well. Since caffeinated beverages such as coffee and colas are diuretics, cut down to one serving a day so you don't lose too much water from your system.

- **Nixed the alcohol.** Sorry. While alcohol can have a place in a long-term healthy diet, if you're trying to lose ten pounds for your college reunion in six weeks, you'll have to stop drinking until then. Not only does alcohol have too many calories to work as part of a 1,000-calorie-a-day crash diet, but it also lowers your metabolism, exactly what you *don't* need when trying to lose weight.

- **Started the meds.** Maria did not want to stay on diet drugs long term, but she did need to weigh in with the agency at least once. So after we'd established her diet and exercise routine, we discussed prescription options. We started her out on a low dose of phentermine. She didn't have any trouble with side effects, so we upped her to the maximum dose after a few days. She kept taking phentermine for two months.

A few weeks later, Maria had dropped seventeen pounds, enough to buy her a bit of slack and a bit of time in the modeling business. Now she maintains just a slightly higher weight with a low-calorie diet and a moderate exercise program. Dropping the weight wasn't easy—crash dieting never is—but it worked for her.

As Maria discovered, if it's really important to you, you can lose ten to fifteen pounds in time for your big event. Just keep two things in mind. First, if you're exercising a lot more than you're used to, you might try judging your success by how the dress you bought for the occasion fits, rather than by the scale. Even cardio exercise can add some lean muscle mass, and muscle weighs more than fat. It also takes up less space, so you'll fit into a smaller dress size even if the scale suggests you won't.

And second, take lots of pictures. You'll want to show them to people once you're done with this diet. Because the important caveat with a crash diet is that you will put some of the weight back on when you take a break after the big day. You've been working hard, so some of it will stay off, and any exercise progress you've made will help you stay slimmer than you would otherwise. But if you've gone much lower than your ideal weight, a few big meals will show immediately.

So relax about it. Enjoy the fact that you looked fabulous, and now work on developing a long-term plan for diet and exercise that suits your goals and lifestyle.

Four

Improving Sexual Performance: His and Hers

EVERYBODY talks about sex these days, but not everyone is getting as much bang out of their banging as they'd like. Walk past a magazine rack, and the headlines scream: Ten Ways to Make Her Moan! Eight Ways to Drive Him Wild in Bed!

We all worry there's something we're not doing right. Is she enjoying herself? Can he last as long as he'd like? For some couples, the stress of trying to do everything perfectly nixes the chances of sex happening at all.

While ads for erectile dysfunction drugs such as Viagra, Levitra, and Cialis have clogged the airwaves during the Super Bowl and inspired much snickering, there is one positive outcome of all the hubbub: Both men and women are more willing to talk about sexual function these days, and seek medical help when they need it. I give that development a big thumbs-up.

One such patient, Brad, came to see me about performance problems. His wife, Erica, had miscarried a few months before, and they were trying to conceive again. They were the typical type-A couple, approaching conception as though they were trying to get into business school. Erica clocked her cycle with two different home ovulation kits, and had constructed a spreadsheet of her basal body temperature to determine the exact moment the odds were in their favor. Brad, on the other hand, was in the midst of launching an IPO with his investment bank, and was spending many of his nights at the office.

When the tests and spreadsheets said it was time, she would e-mail him on his BlackBerry with an urgent message that she was lying in bed, naked and fertile. He'd rush out of a meeting and bolt home to make a baby. But his penis wasn't nearly as excited as his brain. His body couldn't take the pressure of needing to perform *now,* and so he'd lie there in bed, limp.

Many men, because of stress or plumbing trouble or circulatory issues, aren't able to have erections when they'd like to. Others can't last as long as they and their partners would like. Roughly half of women aren't satisfied with their sex lives; up to 30 percent have never had an orgasm, and many women who can give themselves orgasms have trouble achieving them during sex with a partner. Clearly, there are a lot of sexual performance worries out there, enough to keep magazine headline writers cranking out copy about the Nine Orgasm Boosters You Must Try Tonight.

Fortunately, plenty of methods and drugs can help both sexes please themselves and their partners. When we determined that Brad sometimes woke up with erections—that is, he wasn't truly impotent—I suspected he had a classic case of performance anxiety. A dose of Viagra convinced his mind that he *could* have an erection when he needed to and so, soon enough, he did. I'm happy to report that within a few months the couple's own little merger was merrily growing in utero.

While the erectile dysfunction ads have been aimed at men, they've gotten women, and their doctors, talking about female sexual performance as well. I'm starting to see female patients who mention during their annual exams that not everything is as stellar between the sheets as they'd like. So in this chapter I outline a few suggestions for women who don't think they're getting everything out of sex that they can. Almost any woman can have an orgasm during sex, so it's a shame that many women fake it or give up.

Whether you're a man or a woman, when it comes to sex, you don't have to take performance troubles lying down.

For Him

I'm asked daily about the three big impotence drugs on the market—Viagra, Levitra, and Cialis. From rich lawyers to struggling actors, everyone is trying to get the most bang out of their buck, and all have heard that these drugs will make you get harder faster and last longer than you otherwise would. These suspicions are largely true. It doesn't matter if you're driving a Yugo or Ferrari in the sack, even a high-performance machine goes faster with a turbocharger bolted on.

These drugs certainly can help most men with performance problems or worries, from my patient trying to get his wife pregnant to those with third-date jitters. But to understand why and how they work, and what can go wrong with male sexual functioning in general, you first need a basic understanding of male physiology.

When the brain is aroused—be it from touching a partner or thinking about a partner or a stiff breeze—the central nervous system kicks into gear. The epithelial cells in the blood vessels of the sexual organs release nitrous oxide. This triggers the release of a messenger called cyclic GMP, which tells the smooth muscles in the arteries to relax. This causes the blood vessels heading toward the penis to dilate. At the same time, veins that carry blood away from these sensitive organs constrict, so the penis swells up in preparation for sexual activity. In order to reverse the process—and allow blood to flow away from the genitals—the cyclic GMP must be broken down by an enzyme called phosphodiesterase. (The same process affects the clitoris in women.)

These chemicals don't have on-off switches; all three can be in your body at once. It's the balance between them that determines what's going on between your legs. When nitrous oxide and cyclic GMP are floating around in your body in higher concentrations, you're erect. After you ejaculate (or completely lose interest), phosphodiesterase kicks in, and you go limp. If you have too much phosphodiesterase working around in your system from the get-go, you won't get a full erection.

There are a number of reasons that the nitrous oxide/cyclic GMP pathway, and hence, the penis, won't work normally. The most common causes are diabetes and high blood pressure, which narrow your arteries, and stanch blood flow to many places, including your johnson. Any neurologic or vascular problems can also cause difficulties.

But trouble achieving an erection is usually the last symptom of these medical conditions to show up. If you've got diabetes, for instance, you'll know before your penis stops performing. Older men should definitely be screened for heart and vascular troubles, and some medications, such as those for high blood pressure and depression, can cause impotence as well. But in general with young guys, impotence isn't the result of an actual blood vessel problem.

It's also not likely the result of a testosterone deficiency, though many young men blame this hormone for their trouble. Indeed, Brad, my patient who was trying to impregnate his wife, originally came in to ask if he might have this problem. This is a classic response to the Internet search everyone does before heading to the doctor's office. I've learned to hear "low testosterone levels" as code words for trouble with erections, because few men truly suffer from a low testosterone level that has no symptoms besides trouble in the sack.

Testosterone is the hormone that makes men different from women. Low testosterone levels lead to a loss of body hair, breast enlargement, shrunken testicles, and low sexual desire. Men with low desire eventually lose interest in sex, whereas most of the men who ask me about low testosterone levels have plenty of interest in sex; they just can't perform as well as they'd like.

I'm glad patients ask about testosterone though, because one of the *worst* things a guy can do is take testosterone supplements on his own. A young man once came into my office because he was losing the hair on his head and had developed new coarse hair on his back, chest, and arms. He had been using large amounts of an over-the-counter supplement called DHEA, which is popular with men who think it will make them more manly, and with women who use it in hopes of treating menopausal symptoms.

After several months of taking several hundred milligrams of DHEA per day (50 mg is the maximum recommended dose), this young man had an excess amount of testosterone in his system. All the secondary characteristics of maleness were showing up in a bad way, and other than waxing his back, there was not a thing to be done about it. The changes in his body might never be reversed.

Even in older men, low testosterone levels are seldom responsible for poor sexual functioning. About 8 to 10 percent of men over fifty have a testosterone deficiency, and about an equal number have problems with sexual performance, but these are not necessarily the same guys. Most studies show little correlation between the two conditions.

So, if impotence in young men doesn't stem from physical problems, and doesn't involve a testosterone shortage, what on earth, you may ask, is going on?

In fact, good sexual performance depends primarily on what goes on in your brain. This doesn't mean that the problem is "all in your head." Impotence is very real. When there's a problem in the brain, the central nervous system doesn't kick into gear to produce an erection. Pressure, nerves, and stress all keep young men from performing as well as they'd like. Get beyond these, and you've got a better chance of making you and your partner happy.

The first thing to do if you're having trouble achieving erections when you're trying to penetrate your partner, is to see if you're having any erections at all. Can you get one when there's no pressure–for example, do you wake up with a morning erection? If so, then by definition your plumbing works properly.

Even if you don't wake up erect, it's possible you're getting erections during the night. You can test for this by finding a roll of stamps–the kind you lick, not the self-stick variety most places now sell–and wrapping it around your limp shaft before going to bed (you'll have to tape the loose end of the coil). Check the stamps in the morning. If you've experienced tumescence at some point, the stamps will have broken along the perforation.

Most guys trying these tests will discover that they're still physically capable of erections. It's something happening between the brain and the penis that is causing too much stress for physical intimacy. If we're talking about a serious issue like a long-term relationship or marriage on the rocks, then it's time to head for counseling to see what can be done about it. Otherwise, improving performance is just a matter of helping the penis obey the brain.

This brings us back to the topic of Viagra and similar drugs. When the brain is struggling with stress and desire, and can't force the balance of chemical mediators to tip in favor of erection, these drugs help out by inhibiting phosphodiesterase, the chemical we talked about that breaks down cyclic GMP. Without phosphodiesterase inhibiting them, the arteries dilate freely and you get a powerful erection.

While it sounds strange to treat a problem that's in your head with medicine that affects the body, the medicine actually does help the mental part. Brad, the patient who was trying to impregnate his wife, was so eager to conceive that the pressure of trying to copulate was actually preventing it. Most men have this problem at one point or another, and it is tough to get past once it occurs. By taking medications that help you get past this point of anxiety, you can relax, knowing you will be able to achieve full penetration. Once the anxiety is gone, the problem often goes away, too.

Viagra, Levitra, and Cialis don't cause erections by themselves. You have to be turned on to start the chemical cascade that makes blood rush to your loins; these medications just enhance the response. Similarly, once the desire for sex has passed, these medications should only slow the return to normal, not prevent it. This is important to know because on rare occasions, these drugs can lead to an erection that lasts too long—more than an hour or two. When this happens, the blood trapped in the penis can clot, causing permanent damage to the delicate tissues. If this happens, head to the emergency room immediately. In most cases, though, your erection will just be a bit bigger and go away just a little bit slower than usual.

That said, fuller, stiffer, quicker, and longer-lasting erections sound pretty good to most guys, and that's why these drugs are so popular, even among guys without long-term impotence issues. One of my patients loves to talk about an encounter he had with an exotic dancer who happened to sit on his lap after he popped a Viagra. She took his business card and actually called him the next day from the club to gush about his size. Talk about a confidence booster! And often confidence is the most important element in making sex fun for all involved.

So if you've determined that one of these drugs would help you, your next question should be "Which one?" The answer is that there's not much difference between them. Levitra and Viagra both work within a half hour or so, and last for around four hours, though in healthy individuals, sexual response can be enhanced for twelve or more hours. Viagra has to be taken on an empty stomach because fatty foods will inhibit its absorption. Levitra can be taken with or without food.

Cialis is slightly different because it's effective for thirty-six hours. It is an excellent choice for people with impotence caused by medical problems such as diabetes. You can pop one and know you'll have an erection whenever the need for one develops.

However, if you're young and healthy and just suffering from stress-induced impotence, not the impotence that comes from diabetes or high blood pressure, I'd recommend one of the other two drugs. Thirty-six hours is a long time. If you shag successfully on Thursday night after taking Cialis, you are likely to get an erection every time your coworkers bend over on Friday. Some people enjoy that feeling, but given office sexual harassment policies these days, I discourage Cialis use among the young or young at heart.

The Itchy Trigger Finger

Sex, like hosting a good dinner party, is largely a matter of timing, and nobody likes ending the party too soon. A little premature ejaculation can be damaging to self-esteem, confidence, and relationships.

This is a very common problem. When asked, up to a third of men admit to having problems with premature ejaculation on occasion. And since people tend to lie about sexual performance, it's safe to say that the real percentage is probably higher. In fact, almost all men will have trouble with an itchy trigger finger at some point, because the definition of premature ejaculation is that it occurs before you or your partner wants to finish. For some people that's five minutes; for others, it's an hour. For everyone, if you don't work to correct the problem, it can become chronic. And no one wants that.

Thanks to Woody Allen (in *Everything You Always Wanted to Know About Sex . . . But Were Afraid to Ask*), many men believe they should think of baseball when they're sliding too fast toward a home run. Getting your mind off the act, the thinking goes, is as good a way as any of stalling ejaculation.

I'm not a big fan of the baseball technique, though. For starters, there's only so much you can do to forget the writhing body next to you. And if you wanted to count homers at Wrigley Field, you'd be in the bleachers, rather than in bed trying to hit one yourself. If you are looking for a better option, a few techniques can make you last until you and your partner decide it's time to let go.

The first technique is the start-and-stop method. When you feel like the end is near, you stop before that moment of no return and wait it out. This method takes some practice, because your primal instincts at that moment will be urging you to thrust away as fast as you can. Also, your partner may be concentrating on galloping toward her own finish, and she won't want you to stop at that crucial moment. So the two of you will have to work out a method where you stop thrusting, or withdraw and switch to oral or manual sex on her for a minute or so until you regain your bearings.

The second worthwhile technique is The Squeeze. As sexual excitement mounts, but before you're hell-bent toward ejaculation, you pull away and squeeze the base of your shaft with your finger and thumb. This immediately ceases the neurochemical signals that would otherwise push you over the edge. Either you or your partner can do the grabbing, but if it's your partner, make sure she (or he) knows what to do. The last thing you need at this point is more manual stimulation—or pain.

These techniques work well, but there's nothing like stopping in the middle of sex and pinching your shaft to scream "Hello! I have a premature ejaculation problem!" If you're deep into a passionate evening with a new (or newish) partner, you'd probably prefer not to make this so obvious. If that's the case, you can try one of two types of medication to increase your longevity in the sack.

The first are the aforementioned Viagra, Levitra, or Cialis. Not only do these drugs improve the strength of erections, they also delay ejaculation. One dose at least twenty minutes before sex should do the trick.

The second type of drug is antidepressants, which also delay ejaculation, although, clearly, that's not their primary function. Sexual dysfunction is an unfortunate side effect of medications such as Prozac or Lexapro, but for premature ejaculators, this side effect is a welcome one. A single 20-mg dose of Prozac, Lexapro, Celexa, or Paxil taken several hours before sex will delay ejaculation in most men. A onetime dose is unlikely to interfere with your ability to get an erection.

The nice thing about both types of drugs is that they are virtually risk free. The side effects are mild–impotence drugs may cause headache, flushing, and "blue vision" (though I've yet to hear about that one firsthand). The only appreciable side effect from a onetime dose of antidepressants might be some nausea. It's tough to overdose on either (and antidepressants and impotence drugs are safe to use together, if you need them).

The only real risk you face with Viagra and similar drugs is the risk of a rapid drop in blood pressure if you also take certain blood pressure or heart medications that contain nitrates. Nitrates dilate your blood vessels. Viagra, Levitra, and Cialis also dilate your blood vessels. Pop them at the same time, and your blood vessels become too dilated to keep adequate pressure to supply the heart, brain, and other vital organs. This can lead to a heart attack or stroke in some men.

Otherwise, the only risk from drugs that help you get or keep an erection is that, first, you might not be in good enough shape to enjoy the strenuous exercise your newfound virility allows without straining something, and second, you might never reach the finish line. Unfortunately, any technique you use to delay ejaculation gives you a slight risk of not ejaculating at all during that encounter. No harm comes of not coming, but it might not feel so good either.

Supplements for Him

Given the number of men who are worried about performance problems, it's no surprise that you can buy dozens of supplements that tout their erection-boosting power. A few of these supplements work in theory, although the placebo effect for impotence drugs is huge. If you think something will make you erect quicker and longer, it will.

Ginkgo biloba is one popular male supplement. The Chinese used extracts from this tree for centuries, since ginkgo biloba extract dilates blood vessels and reduces the "stickiness" of red blood cells. This improves blood flow to organs, including the genitals. Some preliminary data suggest that ginkgo biloba extract may be effective in aiding memory and concentration as well as sexual dysfunction. Keep in mind that ginkgo acts as a blood thinner, so the greatest risk with this supplement is a chance of bleeding or stroke.

Yohimbine, an extract derived from the West African yohim tree, blocks a receptor that is associated with both libido and blood flow. Unlike most herbal supplements, yohimbine has been synthesized into a prescription drug that can be obtained from a physician. One 5.4-mg tablet, taken three times a day, can improve performance. While this herb can be found over the counter, an FDA study found that eleven of eighteen tested supplements had little or no yohimbine in them. Therefore, while yohimbine might help, you should get a prescription rather than waste money on that over-the-counter variety. You should also keep in mind that anything that works on blood vessels throughout your body can cause serious cardiac side effects in high doses. So stay strictly within the yohimbine dose that your doctor prescribes. This drug should also be avoided by people with kidney disease or psychological disturbances.

L-arginine is an amino acid precursor to nitrous oxide, which (as we talked about above) helps dilate arteries and increase blood flow to the penis. Theoretically, higher levels of l-arginine should mean more nitrous oxide in the sexual organs and a better sexual response. Some studies show no benefit, but at least two trials have shown that l-arginine improves erection strength in over a third of men taking the supplement. This makes it a safe and cheap alternative to Viagra for that lucky third of individuals who respond. The recommended dose is 2–5 grams/day.

DHEA, which caused the back hair problem in the patient I talked about earlier in this chapter, is a precursor to testosterone (and also to estrogen, but its primary effects come from the testosterone side). This means that when you take DHEA, the body metabolizes it into active testosterone. While DHEA can be an effective treatment for anyone who has a true deficiency, there are two problems. First, if you don't have a testosterone deficiency, you don't need any supplementation. Taking a testosterone supplement will just create an overdose of testosterone with complications such as hair loss and shrinking testicles. Second, if you *do* need a supplement, why take DHEA when your doctor can prescribe you actual testosterone to fix the problem?

The last herb that's worth mentioning is the muira puama shrub, native to Brazil and better known as "potency wood." This herb was studied at the Institute of Sexology in France (really). During the study, 262 patients with impotence or a lack of libido took 1 to 1.5 grams per day for two weeks. A little over half reported some benefit. Like ginkgo, yohimbine, and l-arginine, there's little harm to trying this supplement, if only to say you're on potency wood.

Having said all this, I defer to my favorite expert on herbal medications, Dr. Astrid Pujari of the Pujari Center in Seattle, Washington. She's a big fan of herbal medicines, but even she prescribes Viagra before advising a patient to take any of the above supplements. Since none of these herbs come cheap, better to spend your money where it counts.

Ways to Make Her Moan

If you're male and have read the section on improving male sexual performance, you may be tempted to skip the ladies' section of this chapter. That would be a big mistake. While performance issues may create stress in the bedroom, there will be less stress, in general, if she thinks you're a stud. And the best way to make her think you're a stud is to show an interest in making her happy.

Women take longer to warm up than men. A woman's arousal phase starts before she ever undresses. So you need to plant the thought of sex—preferably with you—early. Call her at work and tell her that you can't wait to see her that night. Text message her cell phone all day with updates of what you're planning for the evening. Greet her with a five-dollar bouquet of grocery store flowers "just because." Light some scented candles. Ask about her day. Rub her shoulders. Kiss her hand. Do the dishes. (Seriously. Statistically, men who do more work around the house get more action.) Just don't do this all at the same time, or the same thing all of the time—you want to be smooth, not obvious.

When you're getting ready to have sex, take her clothes off—slowly. Don't dive straight for the genitals. Kiss and touch her everywhere else first. Bonus points for you if you engage in so much foreplay that she's begging you to penetrate her. Whisper in her ear how hot she is. Tell her you want to have sex in position X, Y, or Z because you love looking at her body that way. Ask her if there's anything she'd like to try. If there is, do it. When you're both finished, stay awake for a few minutes to hold her and tell her how much she means to you.

Sure, this takes a bit more time, but happy women want more sex. So think of such generous, caring behavior as a small investment that turns into a big payoff for both of you.

For Her

I started this chapter with notes for men because men are easier when it comes to sex. Get all the pipes working and put their minds at ease, and they're ready to go. Women are more complicated. Up to 30 percent of women have never had an orgasm. Many women who can have orgasms on their own rarely have them during sex with a partner. An astounding half of women have complaints about their sexual functioning. Some of this is related to age—evolution has trained women's bodies to want to make babies, and after menopause, when your body doesn't plan on making more babies, it becomes less interested in sex. Stress, smoking, medications, hypertension, diabetes, and high cholesterol also raise the risk of female sexual dysfunction.

But most causes of dissatisfaction lie squarely between your ears, not between your legs. Women can go through their whole adult lives without learning how to enjoy sex. There's a simple reason for this. Men spend their teenage years masturbating and learning what feels good. Since achieving orgasm is fairly straightforward for guys (thrust away until done), this becomes a simple cycle of wanting another one. With women, however, orgasms involve a combination of the right arousal levels, clitoral stimulation, and a significant psychological component. All the pieces are less likely to be in place the first time you try. If you don't have an orgasm the first time, or the second, or the third, this can turn into a cycle of saying "Why bother?"

For all our differences on the outside, men and women have roughly the same neuro/vascular pathway that causes our sexual organs to start functioning.

Here's how it works. First, women experience the desire for sex. Then they get aroused. When women are aroused, the whole nitrous oxide/cyclic GMP cascade falls into place and blood starts pumping into the vaginal area, particularly into the clitoris. The area swells, just as men get erections. In women, this reaction also causes the vagina to lubricate in preparation for sex. Stimulate the clitoris enough and, as happens when you stimulate the penis enough, you experience that wonderful release of tension known as an orgasm. Then (often more slowly than in men) the resolution phase brings your heartbeat and blood flow back down to normal.

Problems can occur anywhere in the desire, arousal, or orgasm phases. You can have decreased desire, an inability to feel aroused and lubricated because your blood isn't rushing into the labia or clitoris, or you can get plenty aroused but then have trouble achieving orgasm. Women also experience pain during sex at a higher rate than men. Any of these can be labeled "sexual dysfunction," which as you've gathered, is a pretty subjective diagnosis. This isn't like cancer, where there is or isn't a tumor. If sex isn't working well enough for *you*, then you are experiencing sexual dysfunction. Some people are very comfortable with their level of desire and their ability to perform and enjoy sex once or twice a month. Others might feel unsatisfied with sex twice a week.

Like any subjective condition, a lot of women's sexual troubles start in the head. That doesn't mean the trouble isn't real—sex is all about your brain. We're not animals; we need our minds to be on-board for sex to be enjoyable. All the studies on women's sexuality that I reviewed for this chapter had one thing in common: They all demonstrated a huge placebo effect. Whether given a new drug or a sugar pill, women who were told that they were in a study about improving sexual functioning invariably had better sex.

Given that half of women feel they could improve their sex lives, one might think female sexuality would be a ripe subject for investigation. Unfortunately (blame male researchers if you will) there isn't a lot of research out there about women's sexual functioning. This is starting to change, but change comes slowly.

So I've started a more direct form of research: asking women about their feelings on the matter. I've discovered that while many women are not happy with their current or former relationships, most are very happy to talk about it.

It turns out there's an epidemic of faked orgasms out there. Women know—from magazines, TV shows, movies, and so on—that sex is supposed to give them mind-blowing orgasms. They also know that real-life sex does not invariably lead to such a resolution. So rather than tell their partners that they need certain things to achieve an orgasm, or that they haven't actually had one, women start moaning and writhing to (1) soothe the male ego and (2) signal the end of sex for the night.

No man I've spoken to admitted knowing that any woman he'd slept with had faked an orgasm. Most women I've spoken to said they did just that. That means women are doing a hell of a job faking it, and men are quite happy in their state of blissful ignorance.

But this isn't fair to anyone. First, partially satisfying or unsatisfying sex breeds boredom, and boredom leads to cheating or separation. Second, the more you fake, the harder it becomes to tell the truth. You can't just wake up one day and tell your husband that, by the way, the orgasms he thought you were having for the last ten years never happened. Well, you could, but it would create even more problems. So you get trapped by a lie, and the lie puts a barrier into what should be your most honest and intimate relationship.

So rather than faking it, try using your most important sex organ—your mouth. Not for licking, for talking. Communication about sex is never easy, but while a frank discussion may put your guy on the defensive, it opens the door to better sex from then on. If a guy has stuck around for more than one night, he wants you to enjoy sex. The more you like it, the more you're going to want it. Plus, the male ego is built on the premise that each of us is a total stallion in the sack. If you have fun, that shows we're right about how good we are.

Whatever you're trying to tell him, start and end with positive reinforcement. In the middle, suggest something you'd like the gentleman to try. For example: "Honey, sex is great. There's something I'd like you to try (enter request)." Then ooh and aah to show him he's on the right track. Give a puppy a treat for picking up the newspaper, and soon he starts going to the door to wait for the paperboy himself. Likewise, positive reinforcement should have your man asking you for suggestions in no time.

Dr. David Clayton's Guide to Great Sex (for Her)

Before you hit the sheets, there are three things you need to do.

Relax and Enjoy Your Body and Yourself

Women tend to overthink sex. If you worry about what he's thinking, and whether you look like a porn star in the buff, you'll never be able to release your inhibitions and just enjoy yourself. So don't bother. If he's in bed with you, he's probably so grateful that there's nothing more complicated going on in his mind than thinking "Sex . . . good!" And unless you've hopped into bed with an A-list movie star, his body isn't flawless either. Since he's not worrying about his back hair, beer belly, or the acne on his butt, perhaps you can stop obsessing about your stretch marks, cellulite, or the stubble on your thighs. Easier said than done, I know. But one of the reasons I recommend my patients exercise is that hiking, jogging, swimming, and biking are all great ways to start viewing your body as a functional object. You start looking better and better, and you care less and less about how you actually look.

Find a Steady Partner Who Views Women as People and Cares About Your Pleasure

I'm not saying that it's not possible to have mind-blowing sex with a one-night stand. The lack of inhibitions with someone you won't see again is often the reason people get hooked on promiscuity. But a long-term boyfriend, or a husband, has a vested interest in keeping you happy because a happy girlfriend or wife means more sex for him. Also, keep in mind that people who are generous and thoughtful in other areas of life are more likely to be generous and thoughtful in bed. If he talks about himself for the whole first date and never asks about you, sex will also be all about him, and not about your pleasure.

Realize Sex Isn't All or Nothing

Women's magazines, and sometimes men's magazines, too, would have us believe that if the female half of the couple doesn't have an orgasm during every sexual encounter, it's a waste of time. Not true! If you felt sexy and enjoyed yourself and felt closer to your partner, your time was put to good use. Focus on what feels good. For women, having an orgasm takes time, practice, and patience. Pinning all your hopes for the encounter on its end leads to much less satisfying sex.

How to Have an Orgasm

For women, problems can occur anywhere in the desire, arousal, and orgasm phases of sex, or can occur because of pain. If you find sex painful, go to your gynecologist and get checked out. You may have a more serious medical problem that she can help you address.

Or you may just not be lubricating enough. If that's the case, you can pump up the foreplay, or try any of the lubricants available in drugstores to ease things along.

If you feel no pain, but no pleasure either, then you need to work on the desire, arousal, and orgasm phases.

The three are closely intertwined. If you're not sufficiently aroused, you won't have an orgasm. If you don't have an orgasm, you're less likely to desire sex in the future.

My sense is that most younger women who don't have hormonal problems, who aren't on antidepressants, or who aren't worn out from caring for small children don't have real trouble with the desire phase. You may not desire your partner, specifically, if the relationship isn't going well. But if your heart starts racing when you pick up a bodice-ripper novel, or if steamy sex scenes in romantic movies turn you on, you're fine on this front.

Most younger women experience trouble in the arousal phase. That means that they don't get sufficiently aroused to have an orgasm. These women fall into two camps. Some have never had an orgasm. Others can give themselves orgasms during fifteen minutes of private time, but can't have orgasms during sexual intercourse. Both groups *can* have orgasms with a partner, it's just a matter of technique.

Orgasms: What to Do If You've Never Had One

If you've never experienced this whole orgasm thing, you'll need time and patience to start having orgasms during sex. But don't worry. You can succeed. First you need to know how to give yourself an orgasm, then you can teach your partner to give you one.

Next time you've got a few hours alone, take a good look at your body. Make sure you know your anatomy. A mirror can help you get the angle right. For most women, the clitoris–that small (at least on the exterior) nub of flesh at the top point of your labia–is the most sensitive spot. Lie there touching it and see what feels good. What kind of pressure and touch do you like? Add a little lubrication to your finger if this helps. You can use your own lubrication from your vagina, or a commercial variety. Some women like to touch the whole vaginal area and come back to the clitoris from time to time. Others prefer to focus on the sweet spot.

Many women need to focus on a fantasy to push themselves over the edge. Every woman likes something a little different. If you've ever read a romance novel where a sex scene particularly appealed to you, you might picture this scene while you're touching yourself. You can also try reading books of women's fantasies, such as Nancy Friday's *My Secret Garden,* or *Women on Top,* or any of the other collections of erotica available at bookstores. The Internet holds many wonders of this variety. Try visiting sites such as www.Literotica.com for dozens of hot fantasies.

If you read enough stories, you'll likely find one particular variety that knocks your panties off. Concoct your own tale, and try envisioning this while you masturbate. A few attempts should teach you what you like. You may not have an orgasm immediately, but if you relax and keep trying, soon enough, you will. And since much of female sexual functioning is training your mind, once you know you can come, you will come again and again. Next step: trying your new trick with a partner (see below).

Orgasms During Sex

If you've already figured out what makes you feel aroused enough to have an orgasm by yourself, then you're well on your way to getting off with a partner. The trick is to do whatever you were doing to masturbate à deux.

Next time you've got some private time and find yourself excited, pay attention to what you're doing. Do you have a specific fantasy you imagine? Close your eyes and imagine this fantasy while you're having sex. Build toward the climactic moment as your body builds toward climax. Some women feel weird thinking about something other than exactly what's going on while they're having sex, but if you put your partner in a starring role in your fantasy, that should clear up the guilt.

Pay attention to your habits. Do you usually masturbate in a certain position? If you masturbate while lying on your stomach, it may be because you like the way your weight feels pressing your clitoris into your hand. One way to replicate this weight is to use his weight—that is, the missionary position. Experiment with pillows (under your butt or back) and leg placement to get the angle just right. Or you can lie on your stomach with him entering you from behind as you do whatever you do with your hands solo as he thrusts away.

If you masturbate on your back, you may prefer less weight, and the greater control this allows. You can replicate this by climbing on top of him. Experiment with your angle to find the right one. You can also use your hand (or his) to touch your clitoris in the woman-on-top position.

Women who masturbate on their backs may also enjoy getting up on their hands and knees. He enters you doggy style as you engage in some hand action (you may have to lean on a cushion, or the coffee table, for balance). You don't have to use your special position for the whole encounter, just for the few minutes when you're getting close to finishing. Before and after, do whatever you and he both like.

When you masturbate, pay attention to exactly what you're doing with your fingers. If the positions you like allow it, you or he can make the same moves during sex. And keep in mind there's no rule that says you have to have an orgasm while he's penetrating you. If he can replicate your finger action with his hands or tongue, you can get off that way, then have sex in whatever position or style is mutually agreeable. Or you can have sex for a while to get you excited, then have him withdraw for a bit to use his fingers or tongue to get you off, then have him finish inside you.

Teaching him the exact tongue or hand movements that mimic your masturbation style may take some time and communication, but this is truly the gift that keeps giving. You can show him, which he'll find really hot. Or you can give a lot of feedback of the "higher," "harder!" "move to the left a bit," "that's a five, that's an eight, that's an . . . oh my God, a ten!" variety. Positive reinforcement is key. No one likes a schoolmarm in bed, except people who have fantasies about being smacked with rulers, so keep the lessons short, and be sure to reward him with sexual activities he enjoys.

Viagra for Women?

With all the talk of erectile dysfunction drugs, many women wonder when there will be a Viagra for women, or if they can take Viagra and get the same effect. I can't answer the first question, but for the second, the answer is that in premenopausal women, one study showed that women who took Viagra experienced one of three things:

1. They felt nothing different whatsoever,
2. They had the best sex of their lives, or
3. Their clitorises became so sensitive that they couldn't go near men without wincing.

The clitoris becomes engorged and sensitive via the same pathway that makes guys erect, so the clitoris responds to Viagra the same way the penis does. In some women, this is a good thing, as a sensitive clitoris increases the chance of orgasm. In other women, it's a bad thing, because any touch suddenly drives them crazy. While Viagra wasn't designed for women, it's a pretty benign drug, so there's no real downside to trying it. You won't know into which camp you fall until you try.

Both Sexes: Drugs and Their Effect on Sex

Cocaine and ecstasy both increase libido by boosting dopamine and serotonin levels in the brain. The same cascade of neurotransmitters that makes you feel intimate, euphoric, and energized when you take these drugs also makes you want to consummate these feelings in bed. This is usually not a good idea, since when you're baked, you're more likely to "forget" your condom or other birth control method, with all the risks that entails.

But nature has an eye out for you here, working its own strategy of common sense when you lack it. In men, the same neurotransmitters that make you feel happy on cocaine and ecstasy also interfere with your ability to have an erection.

Your body is governed by two main neurosystems: the parasympathetic system, which sends signals telling your body to relax, and the sympathetic nervous system, which sends fight-or-flight adrenaline signals. Erections require "relax" signals. Coke, ecstasy, and crystal meth excite the sympathetic nervous system and cause an adrenaline-like response. Adrenaline responses tell your brain that this is no time to think about sex. So your body stays limp even as your libido soars. When it comes to having sex, party drugs giveth, and party drugs taketh away.

Viagra and other drugs help, but on the whole, sex and party drugs don't couple nearly as well as sober but horny individuals do. Women suffer less from the negative effects of most party drugs than men, since a little lubrication will ease the problem, but they, too, may have trouble finishing up.

Sex and Alcohol

Alcohol lowers inhibitions and increases libido in both sexes. Like party drugs, though, alcohol decreases a man's ability to get and maintain an erection. For chronic and heavy drinkers, alcohol can decrease testicular size and sperm count. In women, high alcohol intake (four or more drinks per day for many years) can stop menstruation, decrease ovarian size, and hence drop the chances of getting pregnant.

These effects in men and women make it less likely that drunks will make babies, but no one should rely on heavy drinking for birth control. No matter how much you drank, you still run a good chance of having a satisfactory sexual encounter—from nature's perspective as well as your own.

Getting More Out of Sex

For both men and women, improving performance is a matter of practice, plumbing, and psychology. Practice is the fun part. Visit your doctor if you suspect plumbing trouble and think you should try one of the performance drugs on the market. But neither practice nor plumbing fixes will lead to great sex if you don't also take care of your brain and your emotions.

So alongside the "Eight Ways to Drive Him Wild in Bed" story, here's one orgasm booster magazines should put on the cover: Great sex, more than anything else, requires great communication. Talk to your partner about what you both like, and what doesn't work. Talk about your insecurities and how you can address them. Then talk about what hot things you're going to try with each other next. While talking about sex is always awkward, life is too short to settle for so-so sex. Opening your mouth is the first step to getting more bang out of your banging. The next steps are up to you.

Five

Pregnancy: Reducing Your Risk

WHEN I was a resident, I often found myself dealing with tragic circumstances: a turn for the worse in an unstable patient, a new and unfavorable diagnosis, a sudden death that sent us hunting for family members to notify. While those cases taught me a lot about being a doctor and a human being, it was also a welcome change to leave those days behind and start treating a group of patients whose medical problems were less likely to be emergencies, and less likely to occur in the middle of the night.

Wherever you practice, though, you still have to tell patients things they don't want to hear. During my first month at the office, I was called into an exam room to break the news to Lilly, a twenty-four-year-old banker, that her pregnancy test turned out positive. She'd just started dating the guy—the liaison in question was on that magical third date, to be specific—and she was desperately hoping it was a false alarm. It took me a long time to tell her, and then answer the questions about her available options.

Babies are wonderful if you want one, but if you don't, an unplanned pregnancy can change your life, and make you face a number of difficult decisions. When Lilly started crying, I made up my mind to preach the Dr. David Clayton Gospel of Pregnancy Prevention to any patient who would sit still long enough to hear it. Here goes:

Young women are pretty much hardwired to make babies. If you're in your early twenties, a year of unprotected sex carries just shy of a 100 percent chance of you getting pregnant. A single act of sex on your most fertile day of the month is 50 percent likely to get you pregnant, 40 percent if you are in your late twenties, and 30 percent in your early thirties. Fertility declines after that, but unprotected sex still leads to conception with shocking regularity.

On the other hand, avoiding an unintended pregnancy isn't rocket science. Ovulation happens only once a month, and ovulation allows for a window of only about twenty-four hours during which you can get pregnant. Add on a few days to allow for the life span of sperm floating around, and you get a maximum window of four to five days a month.

Hormonal contraception methods (particularly birth control pills) and emergency contraception (the "morning-after pill," sold under the name Plan B) are designed to prevent ovulation and implantation, respectively, the two key steps in getting pregnant. Barrier methods, particularly condoms, prevent sperm from getting anywhere near a woman's eggs in the first place.

In short, a woman who is taking the Pill and is having sex with a man wearing a condom has about as much chance of getting pregnant as she does of getting hit by a train—in her bedroom. No egg and no sperm equals no baby. Even if both forms of protection go awry (she missed three Pills and the condom broke) emergency contraception reduces your chances of pregnancy by as much as 90 percent.

Sure, colleagues at the watercooler may tell you a horror story about a cousin's friend's college roommate who was using six methods of birth control and still got pregnant, but there are people who believe the moon landing didn't happen, too. To avoid having a one-night stand end with discussions of child support payments or the gut-wrenching decision to terminate a pregnancy, follow these three simple rules:

Rule #1: Each party takes care of his or her own birth control.
Rule #2: Women: Take the Pill if you can.
Rule #3: Men: Use a condom—and women, insist that they do.

Rule #1: Each Party Takes Care of His or Her Own Birth Control

In an open, trusting, long-term relationship, both parties are on the same page when it comes to family planning. Women who don't want babies right now are quite good about taking care of birth control. But babies aren't always made for good reasons. One of my buddies from college was relying on his girlfriend to take the Pill. One problem with this plan: She wanted a baby; he didn't. Soon, there was an "accident" . . .

Sometimes a guy faced with such an accident decides to stay with the mother. Sometimes it works out, sometimes it doesn't. But if she decides to keep the baby—and guys, you legally have no real say in that matter—you're a father for life, with all that legally entails. And if she doesn't want to keep the baby, and you do, you have no real way to stop her from terminating the pregnancy. And that is a horrible situation as well.

So why risk it? Since my college buddy had his accident, I've recommended that anybody who doesn't want a baby should take responsibility for preventing pregnancy. Guys: If you can't watch her take her Pill, and aren't 100 percent sure she will, skip down to the section on your options. Women: You should insist on a condom anyway. But if, for some reason, you don't, you can pretty much knock out your risk of an unplanned pregnancy by using one of the hormonal birth control methods I'll talk about below.

Rule #2: Women: Take the Pill If You Can

Since the Pill came on the market in the 1960s, millions of women have taken oral contraceptives. They are safe. Even more important: They're a lot easier on your body than giving birth to a nine-pound baby.

Yet somehow the story of the cousin's friend's roommate who had a heart attack on the Pill keeps circulating. I've heard rumors and concerns from my patients about side effects: osteoporosis, a higher risk of cancer, especially breast cancer, weight gain, blood clots, depression, heart disease. Little of this is true. Today's Pills have much lower levels of estrogen-like hormones than the ones women took in the 1960s, and many actually do positive things, such as regulate your cycle, dampen mood swings, reduce acne, and give you lighter, less painful periods. One Pill, Yasmin, even reduces bloating during the cycle. Some women gain weight on the Pill, but a lot of that goes to their breasts. I've yet to hear anyone complain about going from a B cup to a C cup. The Pill does not cause breast cancer, either, so please don't risk an unplanned pregnancy because of that fear.

The most serious possible side effect of birth control pills is an increased risk of blood clots if you're a heavy smoker (fifteen or more cigarettes a day). Even this risk is relatively small for young women, though, compared to your very real risk of pregnancy. For sexually active women who find themselves in situations without condoms handy, a 99 percent reduction in the risk of getting pregnant beats a .01 percent chance of a blood clot. Ask anyone who's dropping out of college to raise a child if she'd prefer that .01 percent chance of a blood clot and see what she says. These percentages are not exaggerated by the way. They're the real numbers.

The Pill also has mental health benefits. You'll always know when you'll get your period—roughly two or three days into the placebo week of a twenty-eight-day pack. Women who aren't on the Pill and who really don't want to be pregnant can go through much mental anguish waiting to see if their cycle will come on time, late, or not at all. That anguish can turn to panic as day twenty-eight becomes day twenty-nine, thirty, thirty-one . . . even though all of these lengths for a monthly cycle are perfectly normal. Why worry? Take the Pill and you won't.

If you're on the Pill, great. If you're not, though, picking from the dozens on the market can be intimidating. Choosing a Pill is a bit like choosing a little black dress. Most are similar in form and function, though some will work better for you than others. You can ask your friends and doctor for advice, and your doctor probably has two or three standbys she always prescribes first. Some people choose Mircette for its headache-fighting power, Yasmin to reduce water-weight gain, or Ortho Tri-Cyclen to battle acne, but it's hard to know how any Pill will work until you try it.

There's no hard-and-fast rule to go by, so most doctors just try you on a couple and find the one that's right for you. This guess-and-test method can be somewhat frustrating if you have a lot of other things to do in your life (and who doesn't?), but consider it an investment and don't give up prematurely. Once you find a Pill you like you can keep taking it for the rest of your childbearing years.

It's very hard to get pregnant on the Pill, even if you miss a day or two. No matter which Pill you are on, these simple rules always apply. If you miss one day, take the forgotten Pill as soon as you remember it. If you miss two days, double up for two days. Any time you start missing pills, you should use a backup method of birth control such as a condom. You should try to take the Pill at the same time every day. Most women take them before they go to bed. My obsessive-compulsive patients double-check in the morning that they've taken the previous night's Pill.

All well and good during weekdays, but here's a catch: On weekends, you might bump into a cute acquaintance at a party. One thing leads to another, and you wind up sleeping at his apartment, not at yours, where your Pills wait by your bedside. What do you do? Those are the days you need your Pills the most.

Here's a trick: Punch your weekend Pills out of the pack on Friday, and keep them in a little zippered coin purse in your handbag. Now if the party goes really well, you're still on schedule. If the party goes incredibly well and you forget all weekend, you can still double up and take these two Pills on Sunday without much chance of getting pregnant. If you're ever in doubt, you can get caught up with one or two Pills, but it's still a good idea to use a backup method just to be on the safe side.

With the Pill, you can also schedule your periods to avoid a big event like your honeymoon. Instead of taking the placebo pills (usually the last seven of the pack), toss them and start a new pack immediately. Voilà, no period. You can do this safely for at least a few months, though I wouldn't go longer than three. To avoid running out of Pills before your next annual checkup, ask your doctor to write the prescription for sixteen or seventeen packs, rather than thirteen. But don't expect your insurance company to cover the extra. Some people can't get their insurance to cover their *heart surgeries.* You'll have to choose if it's worth an extra $100 a year to have fewer periods. An alternative is to go with Seasonale, a birth control pill that is already dosed like this so you don't have to do the thinking on your own.

A side note: You may have read that antibiotics can make the Pill less effective. While it's always a good idea to use a backup method such as a condom, you only need to worry about specific antibiotics used for longer terms (such as tetracycline, commonly prescribed for acne). A short course prescribed for a sinus infection or any other type of transient illness won't cause you to get pregnant if you take your Pills faithfully. So even if you've been treated several times a year for sinus, urinary tract, or any other infections, you shouldn't worry about the safety of your contraception.

Beyond the Pill

Birth control pills are easy to use, convenient, and have been on the market a long time. But they're not for everyone. Some women want hormonal birth control options that they don't have to think about every day. Some women, such as flight attendants, have careers that make taking their Pills at the same time every day a bit difficult. Fortunately, these women have options that are just as effective as the Pill.

The Shot

One alternative to the Pill is the Depo-Provera injection. You receive four shots a year (timed to the first few days of a cycle). Depo-Provera starts working within twenty-four hours and is 99.9 percent effective. If you decide you do want a baby, you'll have to wait a few months for your last shot to clear your system, but you will start ovulating within a year of your last dose, no matter how many doses you had before that.

Depo-Provera has a few downsides. About a third of women taking the shot will have light, irregular bleeding that can happen up to ten days per month. Some women stop menstruating completely, though many people consider this a positive side effect (you can take a pregnancy test if you want to be 100 percent sure that your periods are stopping because of the shot, and not because you're pregnant). Depo-Provera doesn't increase one's risk of breast or ovarian cancer significantly. It slightly *decreases* your risk of endometrial cancer.

The Ring

Another hormonal option is the NuvaRing, a jelly bracelet–looking vaginal suppository that releases the same estrogen and progesterone as other methods of birth control. The small plastic ring is placed in the vagina for three out of every four weeks, and provides the same or a better level of protection as birth control pills.

The Patch

The Ortho Evra Patch delivers the hormones progesterone and estrogen, which are responsible for preventing pregnancy, through the skin. Like the ring, you wear the patch three out of four weeks (on your upper arm, abdomen, back, or butt), and also like the ring, the patch is as or more effective than the Pill when used properly. Both the ring and the patch require care to ensure that they stay where you put them for the whole month. If they are dislodged for more than a few hours, you could become pregnant, so you'll need to use a backup method.

These methods work great to prevent pregnancy, but they're not for everyone. If you've tried several methods and have had trouble with side effects, you still have a few options.

IUDs

Intrauterine devices are small objects placed in the uterus that either release progesterone or are made of a material (copper) that makes the uterus inhospitable to a fertilized egg. Progesterone IUDs have a failure rate of about 1 in 1,000 per year, and copper IUDs have a 19 in 1,000 failure rate. With either, your chances of getting pregnant on any given cycle are slim. Your doctor can insert an IUD during an office visit, and your doctor can remove an IUD in a few minutes as well. The devices last from one to ten years depending on type. Like the Depo-Provera shot, the main downside is irregular bleeding. On very rare occasions IUDs can cause perforation of the uterus or ectopic (tubal) pregnancies. These complications occur in about 1 out of every 3,000 users, which is a fairly low rate, low enough that IUDs are quite popular in Europe (though a bit less so in the United States). In general, IUDs are more popular among women who have finished having children than among those who might want to have children in the near future.

Barrier Methods

If the IUD and hormonal methods don't sound appealing to you, barrier methods provide a decent level of protection against pregnancy, particularly as you get better at using them. The diaphragm and cervical cap both work by blocking sperm from entering the uterus (and kill the sperm, if you add spermicides). Both are side-effect free—no manipulating your hormones—but their failure rates, 3 to 17 percent, are a bit intimidating. If you decide to use a diaphragm or cervical cap, you'll need to be fitted by your gynecologist. Then you'll need a few quick lessons from your gynecologist on how to use them. The 17 percent failure rate is mainly from folks who just shove the diaphragm in and trust it will do its job. (Hint: It's a *bit* more complicated than that—so pay attention and practice.)

Female Condoms

Another barrier method was launched to much hype a few years ago. These condoms are just what they sound like—a barrier that goes inside the vagina instead of on the penis—and they provide protection the same way male condoms do. Female condoms let women exercise control over STD and pregnancy prevention, but they have two drawbacks. First, they have a slightly higher failure rate than male condoms, and second, almost a third of women give up on female condoms after a few months. A lot of folks, apparently, do not like how female condoms feel. If you're trying to convince a guy to use a male condom, you might try a female condom and see if he stops complaining about his own rubber thereafter.

Rule #3: Men: Use a Condom—and Women, Insist That They Do

The male condom is the best barrier method available. It protects against both pregnancy and STDs. Since waiting to have sex long enough to verify that both parties are disease-free and using a hormonal birth control method is a trying experience for many people, using a condom is a no-brainer. Except . . .

> "I don't like the way they feel."
>
> "I can't get an erection with a condom."
>
> "I can't come when I'm wearing a condom."
>
> "I didn't want to ask if he had one, because even though we were both naked and in bed, I didn't want him to think I was that kind of girl."
>
> "It isn't natural."
>
> "We never have a condom handy when the moment is right. What are we going to do, put on our clothes and go to the drugstore?"
>
> "I'm allergic to condoms."
>
> "My boyfriend/man of the moment doesn't like condoms."

Both parties may have no problem asking for a 25 percent raise, or telling the client that the project will run them $1 million a month, but somehow, when it comes to protecting against STDs and pregnancy, they are prisoners of circumstance. The excuses tumble out like coins from a slot machine. Guys: Yes, a condom doesn't feel as good as just being inside her, but trust me, if you don't know for sure that she's on the Pill or using another method, an unplanned pregnancy doesn't feel so hot either. Someday you'll meet someone you'll want to have sex with for months—*or years*—and you can ditch the condoms. And that special woman will be much happier if you don't have any previous tots entitled to a percentage of your paycheck.

Of course, guys aren't the only half of a couple who can take responsibility for bringing and using condoms. Women can keep a few in their handbags (perhaps in that same coin purse with the weekend Pills). You can tell a guy it's too bad you'll just have to cuddle instead if he balks at wearing one. You can pull one out at the right time and simply start rolling it on him (pinch the tip to leave a bit of space, then roll on down the shaft) without making a big deal about it. When one party decides to act responsibly, the other party tends to go along—and once the condom's on, he's unlikely to take it *off.*

That said, I live in the real world. If you aren't going to use a condom, there are two other methods you can use to reduce the chances that sperm and egg will meet.

Pull Out

Yes, withdrawal, also known as coitus interruptus. Shortly before you ejaculate, you can pull out and use your hand (or hers) to push yourself over the edge. Some of my patients claim this is a more natural method of birth control; however, pulling out means no mutual orgasms, and requires an incredible amount of self-control, not to mention a sexual partner who's comfortable with the mess you're going to make on her stomach, thighs, and nice clean sheets.

But those are the downsides. The upside is that pulling out does work. It's a common misconception that the little bit of preejaculatory fluid that dribbles out of the penis actually contains sperm. However, the scant medical research on the topic shows that there's no sperm in there, and hence no risk of getting pregnant without a real ejaculation. So if you're not going to use a condom, pulling out does dramatically reduce your risks. If you want to come inside her, and still can't be bothered with condoms, make sure you only complete the act during her least fertile days—during or right before her period. Don't know her well enough to ask when that is? Now we're back to "use a condom."

Masturbate Beforehand

One of my med school buddies always tried to convince me that masturbating before sex was a good way to get rid of all the sperm, in case the condom broke or you "forgot." So I did the research and found out that he was onto something. One ejaculation reduces the sperm count in a subsequent ejaculation by 30 percent. Now, 70 percent of your swimmers are still enough to impregnate a woman—you do release millions, after all—but it's a start. A second round of masturbation will cut down from that 70 percent. Then the next time . . .

As you can see, this isn't a great method. If your date stops by beforehand and finds you ensconced with your Jenna Jameson photos, she may think differently about you. And if you masturbate three or even four times before your date, you might be sore, not to mention not in the mood—or even capable of achieving an erection—when it's time to have sex with your partner. Wearing a condom sounds a lot more pleasant to me than risking carpal tunnel syndrome or temporary impotence. But if the condom stays in the car or your partner feigns an allergy, this method is better than nothing.

Less Effective Techniques

The birth control methods currently on the market work remarkably well to prevent pregnancy. A few other methods work much less well.

Perhaps, for example, you know a devoutly religious couple that touts "periodic abstinence"—not having sex on her most fertile days. Perhaps you've also noticed that these people tend to have large numbers of children. This is because the rhythm method, just like the pulling-out method, requires a lot of self-control. A woman can only get pregnant within about twenty-four hours of her ovary releasing an egg. But sperm can survive inside her for five or six days before that. So we're looking at avoiding sex on days eight through fifteen of her cycle (counted from the start of her last period). But what if she doesn't ovulate on the fourteenth day? What if her ovaries wait until day fifteen, sixteen, or seventeen? Soon we're up to a two-week period of abstinence. Since most people cut back on sex during menstruation (days one to five or even seven), that leaves just one week a month to go wild. While this is good to know if the condom breaks during the last week of her cycle—that is, there's no real reason to be alarmed—most couples can't wait for one week out of every four just to have sex. That's what causes those families of children spaced every year.

Breast-feeding is also not a good method of birth control. I recently met a nice couple who came to New York from India after the husband was accepted to grad school. They'd already had one child in India, and weren't looking to have more until he was done with school and gainfully employed. At the time, she had been breast-feeding for about nine months or so, and they were under the impression that there was no risk of pregnancy this soon after the baby was born. But then she started feeling a familiar sense of fatigue and morning sickness. They went to their doctor's office, mystified. The explanation: Breast-feeding does suppress ovulation, but not reliably, and not for long. Obviously, you can get pregnant within a year after giving birth, even if you are still nursing.

What to Do When the Condom Breaks

In the wee hours of a Sunday morning recently, a patient I'll call Jessica phoned me, panicked. It was day fourteen of her cycle, Jessica said, and the condom broke. She wanted to know what to do. So I asked for the number of her local pharmacy. She looked it up, called me back, and I called in a prescription for Plan B, a brand of emergency contraception. As the ad for Preven, another brand of emergency contraception that's no longer being manufactured, used to say, "The condom broke . . . but my life stayed intact." Once a ridiculously well-kept secret, emergency contraception, or the "morning-after pill," can reduce your risk of getting pregnant by 75 to 90 percent on your most fertile days by preventing you from ovulating, or keeping a fertilized egg from implanting.

It's always possible that the morning-after pill will be available over the counter someday, but currently you need a prescription for Plan B. You take one dose as soon as you can fill the prescription, then the other twelve hours later.

You can also make a morning-after pill yourself if you have birth control pills sitting around the house (though if you do, you should be taking them, and not needing morning-after pills in the first place). Here are a few examples for do-it-yourself types:

- Ovral, Ogestrel (high-progesterone pills) : two tablets, then two tablets twelve hours later
- Lo/Ovral, Low-Ogestrel, Levlen, Levora, Nordette: four tablets, then four tablets twelve hours later
- Alesse, Aviane, Lessina, Levlite: five tablets, then five tablets twelve hours later

Some very low hormone dose Pills such as Ovrette require dosages of twenty pills or more to have a morning-after pill effect. Unless you enjoy swallowing pills, it's a lot easier to ask your doctor to write you a just-in-case Plan B prescription next time you're at her office. If you don't have a doctor you can call, you can get the names and phone numbers of emergency contraception providers near you by calling the hotline 1-888-NOT-2-LATE. You can call the nearest Planned Parenthood at 1-800-230-PLAN. You can also go online to www.GetThePill.com and for $24.95, a doctor will call in a prescription (have your pharmacy's number handy when you go to the Web site).

It's tough to see why anybody wouldn't take emergency contraception after an accident. The pills are readily available, so not having them on hand is no longer a good excuse. Most of the time, what I hear is that women don't know much about emergency contraception, and worry about its safety.

I can assure you that emergency contraceptive pills are very safe. So far only a handful of possibly related blood clots have been reported in medical journals, out of all the pills ever prescribed. Even for people with a history of blood clots or liver disease (questions your doctor may ask before prescribing Plan B), using the morning-after pill is still statistically safer than going into the high-risk pregnancies that these folks often have. If you are healthy, the morning-after pill may make you nauseous, and will probably cause you to have a period sooner than otherwise, but that's about it. Buy some Dramamine or ask your doctor for an antiemetic, eat some saltines, and you'll be fine. Remember, risks are relative. Even if Plan B isn't 100 percent side-effect free, you've got to weigh the side effects of a few birth control pills against the very real risk of an unplanned pregnancy.

Most important: If you are already pregnant from an encounter earlier in the month, or you're one of the few for whom the medicine doesn't work, emergency contraception will not harm your baby. Neither will conventional birth control pills. That's a lot more than can be said of many things pregnant women do to their bodies.

How to Know If You're Pregnant

Easy: You take a test. But you have to wait at least a week after the possible conception for even the most sensitive pregnancy tests to register positive. While every gynecologist has a story of a patient who just "knew" from day one she was pregnant, I believe these stories are based on 20/20 hindsight (it's easy to say you "knew" once the test turns out positive). Typical pregnancy tests require at least five to seven days after conception to turn reliably positive, because they rely on a surge in the hormone beta-HCG, which is produced by a viable embryo. If the condom breaks on day fourteen, and you take a pregnancy test on day sixteen, the results will be meaningless. One large, well-designed study of women age twenty-one to forty-two using a urine pregnancy test found these accuracy rates:

Two days before the first day of the missed period: 79 percent accurate
The first day of the missed period: 90 percent
Seven days after: 97 percent
Eleven days after: 100 percent

So when it comes to pregnancy, you just won't know for sure if you are or aren't until at least a week and maybe two to three weeks after the act of intercourse.

That's a tough wait. A possible unplanned pregnancy has a way of seizing hold of your brain until you can think of nothing else. I've had calls from patients analyzing every stomach twinge, every bit of dizziness, every possible pain in their breasts as symptoms of pregnancy. But here's something to put your mind at ease, at least for a while. It takes a few weeks after conception for pregnancy hormones to start giving you the traditional symptoms of morning sickness or general lethargy. Before a missed period, any traditional pregnancy symptoms you are experiencing are likely something you ate, guilt, paranoia—or PMS.

Another thought, which should be obvious: If you get your period, a real period, not just spotting after rough sex, you're highly unlikely to be pregnant. Yet when it comes to pregnancy, even the obvious gets lost in the shuffle. One very intelligent woman I know allowed a colleague to convince her that she could be pregnant even though she was having her period *and* was on the Pill, just because she'd been throwing up for a day. Of course, she panicked and insisted on coming in for a pregnancy test immediately. We complied—it never hurts to take a test. But once it came up negative, the nausea disappeared like a snickering coworker into a cubicle.

If you miss a period or just want the assurance of knowing one way or the other, you can buy pregnancy tests quite easily online these days. No need to ask that acne-faced seventeen-year-old drugstore clerk to unlock the glass case for you. Do a Google search on "pregnancy tests" and you'll find plenty. Online pregnancy test providers will ship you the tests, overnight if you want, and in unmarked packages. Do yourself a favor and buy two. If you get nervous and make a mistake that produces an ambivalent stripe or color, you'll be happy to have a backup sitting right by.

Another note: If you do miss a period, *please* take a pregnancy test; you'll need to know right away so you can figure out your next step. Denial won't stop a pregnancy once it's under way. A woman I know recently informed me that her daughter had just given birth "spontaneously" with no warning whatsoever. I never figured out the details—obesity? baggy sweaters? nine months of coincidentally missed periods?—but the whole family needed a shrink more than they needed me.

If You Are Pregnant and Don't Want to Be

I hope no one who's read the first section of this chapter ever needs to read this section. If you and your partner find out you're pregnant, and you decide that you cannot have a baby, abortion remains a legal option. In the first trimester, abortions are fairly safe and easy. But they're never easy on your psyche, and that's important to keep in mind. Unfortunately, because abortion is an available option, some women (and more men) are not as careful with birth control as they should be. For guys, this is an especially bad strategy. You can't force her to have an abortion, after all, and if your partner decides to have your baby, you are facing eighteen years of child support payments whether you stay with the mother or not. And for women, for all the rhetoric about choice, this is not a fun choice, and it's likely one you'll ponder for the rest of your life. It's far easier to take the Pill and use a condom and never wind up in this situation.

But if you do . . . Most abortions are performed surgically by gynecologists in the first or second trimester of pregnancy. First trimester abortions are minor procedures done at the office, and usually take less than an hour. In the most commonly performed procedure, the doctor will dilate your cervix with a small instrument and insert a suction catheter into the uterus. Your doctor will scrape your endometrial lining and suction the area to remove any viable tissue, then she'll withdraw the catheter. The mortality rate during this procedure is around 1 in 100,000, and it's safest when performed at around eight weeks.

If you don't want a surgical abortion, in the first trimester you can also have a "medical" (drug-based) abortion. You take a series of two pills over two days. The first dose, either methotrexate or mifepristone (formerly known as RU-486), is followed by a dose of misoprostol; the combination of the two drugs causes a complete expulsion of everything in the uterus over the first couple days. If the drug combo fails for some reason, the fetus will likely have serious birth defects, so any failed attempt must be followed by a surgical abortion. Medical abortions have a mortality rate of about one death per million, and are 95 percent effective within the first forty-nine days after your missed period.

While many people think abortions are only done at abortion clinics surrounded by pro-life picketers, in fact many ob/gyns perform these procedures in their offices, just as they would perform any other type of office procedure. If you live in a reasonable-size city, you can look in the phone book to see who offers these services; you'll likely find a few pages of ads. Or you can call around to ob/gyns in your area and ask. If you already have a gynecologist, call the office to ask her for a referral, or ask if she does these procedures herself.

But don't forget about your emotional state as you're paging through the phone book. Even if you are totally committed to terminating an unexpected pregnancy, the decision is always an emotional roller coaster. One of my patients, Anne, was going through some tough times with her recent divorce, and sought solace through antidepressant medication and a therapist, both of which were good ideas, and in the arms of three men over the course of a month, which turned out not to be such a great idea. She wasn't thinking about pregnancy, she explained later, because the liaisons–her ex-husband, a longtime friend, and a one-night stand–didn't "count." However, they all started to count a lot more when she found out that she was pregnant. She had no idea who was the father, and none of the men seemed particularly interested in raising a baby. So an agonizing week later, Anne made her appointment and had the pregnancy terminated. Unfortunately, none of the potential fathers were by her side, nor had she lined up any support from family or friends. She went home crying and couldn't stop. The post-termination stress wound up exacerbating her depression so badly that she ended up voluntarily committing herself, and spent two days in a mental hospital recovering.

The takeaway from this story is that before you even consider having an abortion, surround yourself with people who will support your decision and be with you for some time afterward. If your partner won't step up to the plate, or you don't think you can tell him, find a friend or family member to lean on. If you can't go to a friend or family member, ask your gynecologist to refer you to a counselor or therapist. Some women's health care centers also have counselors on staff. That's a side benefit that's worth looking into as you page through the phone book.

If you're concerned about privacy, flip ahead to the last chapter of this book for advice on who can see your medical records and whether anyone will be able to find out whether you had an abortion.

If You Do Want to Have Babies Someday

Many women who don't want babies now do want to have them someday. In my practice, I'm amazed how women fall into two categories: those who don't want to get pregnant but do, and those who desperately want a child but can't conceive. Many infertility cases are age-related. You can conceive up until menopause, but it gets much harder along the way. According to the American Society for Reproductive Medicine, one third of women over age thirty-five have trouble conceiving, and two thirds of women over age forty have fertility problems. I know it's not fair. Despite the fact that sperm gets less healthy as men age, time favors men over women when it comes to conception. Men can father children with their trophy wives well into their seventies, but women realistically need to be thinking about childbearing before it gets too late.

One thing you can do to slow down the clock a bit is to stay healthy. Don't smoke. Keep yourself at a healthy weight. Don't drink more than one alcoholic beverage or so a day, and don't use illegal drugs. You should also ask your doctor to test you for various STDs. Gonorrhea and chlamydia (which often goes undetected) can affect fertility, so get screened annually.

You should also keep in mind that the reduction in fertility rates among older women means that you're less likely to conceive on any one cycle. So if you're trying to have a baby, don't be surprised or disappointed if it doesn't happen the first month. You may have to keep trying. But if you've been trying for a year with no success, consult your gynecologist to look into different options.

Birth Control—Just Do It

Almost half of pregnancies in this country are unintended. Not all of those unintended babies are being born to teenagers who don't know any better, which means a lot of people who *should* know better are causing needless turmoil for themselves and their partners by "forgetting" to think about birth control and emergency contraception until it's too late.

There are enough methods of birth control on the market that no one need face an unintended pregnancy. If you're a sexually active woman, there's no excuse for not finding a gynecologist and having a talk about what method is best for you. If you can't afford a private practitioner, or don't have insurance, try a Planned Parenthood in your area or a women's health care clinic. Your ob/gyn will likely tell you that birth control pills work wonderfully for most people. If you have trouble remembering daily pills, you can choose another method such as the patch, the shot, or the ring—whatever fits your lifestyle. Even if you discover that you can't use a hormonal method of birth control, barrier methods such as the diaphragm or female condom give you decent protection against pregnancy. While you're at the gynecologist, ask for an advance prescription for Plan B that you can fill now and take in case you have an emergency.

Men have just as much responsibility for ensuring that a hook-up doesn't end with a discussion of child support payments. If you don't have any condoms in your wallet or apartment, *now* would be a good time to go buy some. If you're embarrassed to shop for them because you'll have to face the drugstore clerk, don't be. The drugstore clerk just sold someone adult undergarments and hemorrhoid cream. The drugstore clerk does not care that you're buying condoms. But if you are worried, go online to some place like drugstore.com and have them shipped.

Once you're prepared, keep in mind that condoms don't prevent pregnancy if you don't use them. When things are heating up, before you go in, bring it out and put it on. Don't bother explaining or saying anything beyond how much you can't wait to be inside her. If the relationship develops, after you both get tested for STDs and verify that she's using a hormonal or effective barrier birth control method, then you can go bare. Until then, a condom is your best friend.

The bottom line is that both partners have plenty of methods and plenty of time to prevent pregnancy. While it's possible to terminate a pregnancy, you never want to be in the position where you need to make that choice. So, take a few minutes to plan ahead so a drunken night of passion doesn't screw up the rest of your life.

Six

STDs:
What You Can Catch
and How Not to Catch It

ONE of my first patients in New York was a young man who came in wanting to see, specifically, a male doctor. That tipped me off—whenever a guy asks for a male doctor, the conversation is bound to come around to his genitalia.

Sure enough, this man told me he had slept with a new woman two days earlier. He was worried he might have caught something, because he had some redness and swelling. So we brought him into the exam room. Then he took off his pants, and I almost fell off my stool. His entire package was one swollen, oozing mess. You could barely figure out which part was his penis. Dumbfounded, I asked what happened. He confessed that after having sex with this woman, he became so concerned about catching a disease that he took a loofah and some rubbing alcohol and tried to scrub the germs away.

I told him we couldn't be sure he hadn't picked up anything until we ran some tests, but it was unlikely she could have done more harm to him than his paranoia had made him do to himself.

Over time, and after seeing many patients like Loofah Guy, I've realized something about sexually transmitted diseases (STDs): Plenty of people have them—an estimated 22 percent of the population is walking around with herpes—but there are just as many people who think they've contracted something and haven't.

I blame schools for this paranoia. Today's young professionals were the good students who watched health class films on "social diseases" with only moderate snickering. We grew up during the AIDS crisis of the 1980s, and had public health nags drill into our heads that one unprotected sexual encounter could lead to a slow, painful death for you, your partners, and your future children.

No wonder people panic. Most of my patients are sexually active; many of them sleep with people of the same sex. And at some point, a good number of these intelligent people will go to their doctors in a panic because they're convinced they've caught something and their lives are over. They've spent the night before their appointment locked in the bathroom staring at their genitalia in a mirror, trying to divine the meaning of each bump like soothsayers looking through the entrails of a sheep. They've moved their laptops to where no one can see, and have been Google searching for pictures of herpetic lesions and syphilitic chancres. It doesn't matter if they're in committed relationships or promiscuous. In fact, the monogamous have more questions than the promiscuous, because the promiscuous have already figured out what I'm about to tell you.

While I'm glad to see people seeking help when they're concerned, and I encourage it, there's a lot of misplaced worry about STDs. For starters, while you can catch something from unprotected, or even protected, sex, the risk is fairly low from any one encounter with a partner who doesn't sell sex or drugs for a living.

Second, many of the pimples and bumps people worry about are perfectly normal. Even acute symptoms, such as pain during urination or itching, can be caused by common bacterial or yeast infections, not just STDs.

Third, if you *have* caught an STD, many, such as gonorrhea and chlamydia, are curable with a short course of antibiotics. Even those that aren't curable—such as herpes—are treatable these days with drugs that suppress outbreaks and reduce your chances of passing the disease to others. Human papilloma virus (HPV), which most sexually active women contract at some point, is connected to cervical cancer. However, it often goes away by itself, and with regular screening by a gynecologist the precancerous cells can often be destroyed before they cause problems. Even HIV can be treated with a number of drugs that stop or slow its progression, so the diagnosis is no longer an immediate death sentence.

I won't pretend that there aren't serious health and quality-of-life issues associated with STDs like herpes. An HIV infection will require a lifetime of treatment with multiple drugs that have some serious and occasionally nasty side effects. But even people with incurable STDs live full and productive lives in this country.

So I hope everyone reading this chapter will calm down a bit about STDs. You might not have anything, and if you do, your doctor will help you take care of it. While you may be embarrassed to seek medical attention, remember, like my patient, you're not going to be able to treat STDs yourself by attacking your private parts with a loofah.

If you're too embarrassed to see your own doctor, most towns have walk-in clinics that deal with STDs all the time. They won't judge you. Seriously. Come in at noon and you could be gonorrhea infection number four for the day. The only reason anyone will judge you is if you knowingly pass an STD to someone else. Now *that* is a contemptible thing to do.

A Primer for the Uninitiated

The problems we're talking about in this chapter are caused by organisms that fall into several categories: viruses, bacteria, parasites, and fungi. If you skipped science class in school because it bored you, skip to the prevention section below, but for any budding infectious disease specialists, here are the details:

DNA and RNA are the basic genetic codes of organisms. DNA is the blueprint; RNA is the construction crew that translates the

DNA, then assembles the amino acids into complex proteins that link together into structures.

Viruses are protein-wrapped strands of DNA or RNA that have only one purpose in life: replication. Viruses have just enough genetic code to copy themselves, so they need to invade other cells—yours—to come up with the rest. When you're exposed to a virus, it latches on to your cells, gets inside, and destroys the cells in the process of copying itself. While this sounds ominous, it actually happens all the time (for instance, when you catch a cold). Usually your immune system identifies the virus and kills it before it does much damage.

Bacteria are more complicated. These single-celled organisms can live peacefully in the body. For instance, your skin right now is covered with staphylococci and other bacteria that do not usually cause problems or infections. Problems arise when the bacteria replicate and start competing with your cells. If you get a scrape or cut, for instance, the staphylococcal bacteria can enter your body, multiply, and cause an infection.

Parasites are either tiny and simple, like chlamydia, or complex, like leeches, but they all need hosts to survive. Chlamydia needs to be inside one of your cells, and a leech needs to suck on your blood. These parasites aren't trying to kill you, though. If they do, they die as well. For this reason, most parasites, including leeches and intestinal parasites, might make you ill or terribly ill, but are rarely lethal.

Fungi and **yeast** are two forms of the same multicellular organism; their cells branch onto one another either in a jumble like a yeast infection or in a complex pattern like a mushroom. Fungi are all around us. They wait to find nice warm moist places, then they grow.

We are exposed to many of these organisms every day. We keep them at bay with basic hygiene and solid immune systems. The point of this chapter, though, is what happens when they breach our defenses. So let's move on.

Prevention

I know many people poring over this chapter have had sex with a new partner recently and have now become paranoid about what germs and viruses jumped under the beach blanket with them. More on that in a minute. First, a dose of prevention can prevent much anxious rumination later.

Before You Have Sex with a New Partner

The best way to ease your mind about STDs is to look at yourself before you think you've caught anything. Get to know your body below the waistline. Ladies, a handheld mirror will improve your angle. Often, people don't know what their equipment looks like until the morning after a one-night stand, when that little pimple they've never noticed leaps out in full color. Everyone's genital skin has imperfections, and you can quell a lot of concern by knowing those imperfections have always been there. Grab a bright light and focus on any bumps, irregular skin surfaces, or areas where the texture is different from the surrounding skin. See what the hair follicles look like, if any of them have clogged up and created pimples, and notice your skin's natural coloring.

For men, the most common red herring is the small "pearly penile papules" that line the edge of the prepuce, or head of the penis. This row of tiny translucent bumps is a normal feature of the glans penis. If you have it, make a note of it, so you don't think the bumps are a precursor for herpes later on. Once you've got your basic layout scoped, you'll be better prepared to compare the postsex appearance of any new features to the graphic pictures you find on the Internet.

Common Sense

As with pregnancy prevention, the best way to prevent STDs is through abstinence. You can't catch an STD if you don't have intimate sexual contact with someone. If you are going to have sex, STD prevention still isn't rocket science. Also, like pregnancy prevention, it's routinely ignored by people who should know better.

Before we even get to the lecture about using condoms, three simple actions will lower your risk of discomfort and itchiness:

1. **KNOW.** Get to know your partners before having sex. Someone you've dated for several months has more invested in you and your health than someone you ordered up from an escort service. If you ask a one-night stand whether he's been tested for STDs recently, he may lie and tell you yes. A boyfriend or girlfriend, on the other hand, might agree to get tested with you.
2. **LIMIT.** Keep your total number of partners in check. There's no magic number. Under ten won't keep you clean, and over ten won't guarantee an infection, but it helps to imagine whether your future spouse would cringe if you shared the correct count.
3. **LOOK.** Take a good look at your partner. Not in the eyes. Between the legs. I'm not advocating a thorough exam, but if you can pull it off, keeping the lights on long enough to notice whether the person has sores or lesions can save you a host of trouble later.

Condoms

As for condoms, this is an easy one. If you don't know whether your partner has an STD, and you'd prefer not to catch one, wearing a condom isn't negotiable.

Sure, condoms aren't perfect. Sometimes they break. Sometimes they don't cover all the warm, wet tissue in which germs thrive, so you can be exposed to herpes or HPV even if you are wearing a condom. But condoms are much better than nothing, and are very effective in preventing transmission of the more serious diseases such as HIV, hepatitis, and even gonorrhea and chlamydia.

Don't worry about picking the right condom. Things like fit and feel are a matter of personal preference, and can provide ongoing fun for you and your partners as you try different ones. Given the myriad choices, and given how little you'd like to stand in front of the display rack at the drugstore, zero in on what matters: protection.

Latex condoms offer the best protection against HIV, hepatitis, syphilis, herpes, warts, chlamydia, and gonorrhea. If you have trouble with latex, polyurethane condoms also offer good protection against STDs, and some people prefer the thinner, more transparent feel of these condoms (many others, however, don't like their higher price). Avoid sheepskin or "natural" condoms, since their permeability makes them a poor choice for preventing STDs. If you're going to the trouble of wearing a condom, you want one that does its job.

Regardless of the condom you choose, here's a little factoid that gets lost in the rush to penetration: Condoms don't work if you don't use them.

If you're leaping into bed with someone new, and he or she is willing to go bare, this should be a huge red flag. No matter how special the occasion is, or how he swears up and down that he's never done anything like this, someone who is willing to plunge in sans protection is more likely to be carrying something than someone who isn't. If your partner wants to go bare, the sobering 22 percent prevalence of herpes in the population is likely a lot higher where you are right now.

More food for thought: You are most at risk of catching an STD in the first three months of a new sexual relationship. Diseases are most contagious right after they take root in the body. If the person you're sleeping with was recently exposed to HPV, herpes, or even HIV in his or her last relationship, he or she will be more likely to expose you in the early days of your new relationship.

So in the beginning, insist on the condom or slow down. *Way* down. Put your clothes back on and say you'll cuddle instead. That ought to change your partner's mind.

Spermicides

Unlike condoms, spermicides are a mixed bag. While spermicides do prevent pregnancy, there's some evidence linking nonoxynol-9, the most commonly used spermicide, with a higher incidence of STDs such as gonorrhea and chlamydia. This is likely because spermicides can cause irritation in both sexes, increasing the ability of bacteria and viruses to penetrate the skin. Besides, spermicides kill sperm (hence the name) *not* STD organisms. If you're using condoms as a method of birth control, then in the balance it makes sense to use a condom combined with spermicide. But if you and your partner are primarily concerned about STDs, and you're using a hormonal contraceptive or an IUD, skip the nonoxynol-9.

Vaccines

Unfortunately, using condoms and abstaining from sex with infected partners are the only ways to avoid most STDs. That's not the case, however, with hepatitis A and B, for which you can be vaccinated.

Many viruses cause hepatitis, which means they directly attack the liver. The three most common in developed countries are A, B, and C, and while they technically do the same kind of damage to the liver, they are transmitted in different ways.

Hepatitis A is transmitted through the intestinal tract, meaning it's got to come out of someone's rear end and go into your mouth in order for you to catch it. This makes the disease primarily of concern to those traveling to countries with lousy sanitation, those eating in restaurants where workers don't wash their hands, or those engaging in oral-anal sexual practices. The virus can survive for days on surfaces and is resistant to most cleaners and heat. Once ingested, it enters the intestinal tract and heads straight for the liver, where it invades liver cells and destroys them.

About four weeks after exposure, you'll notice vague, flulike symptoms, loss of appetite, and vomiting. Severe hepatitis can cause bilirubin, the pigment made in the liver that turns stool brown, to leak into the bloodstream. This turns your urine brown, your eyes yellow, and your stools gray or white. There's no real treatment other than close monitoring by your doctor to prevent complications. Some people's livers can fail from hepatitis, but most people get better over the next one to six months.

Still, that can be a very unpleasant six months. So why risk it? There's a vaccine readily available at your doctor's office or a travel clinic, and after a booster in six to twelve months, you can forget worrying about hepatitis A again. So if you're at risk, get the vaccine.

Hepatitis B, unlike hepatitis A, is transmitted by sexual contact and blood. The virus enters through the genital tract or an open sore or wound, and again goes straight for the liver. Symptoms are the same as for hepatitis A, and occur one to six months after exposure.

There are two pieces of good news about hepatitis B. Most people who get it never know it, because their immune systems eradicate the virus and they regain their health and become completely immune from catching it again. In this case, carriers who are immune can't and won't transmit it to others. The second bit of good news is that there is also a three-shot series of vaccine that can give you total immunity. If you haven't already gotten the vaccine there's no reason not to, especially when you consider the bad news. About one in ten hepatitis B patients has a chronic version of the disease. A hepatitis B patient's liver can slowly deteriorate until she develops cirrhosis or cancer.

Hepatitis C is transmitted through blood, not through sexual contact, unless your sexual contact involves blood. There is no vaccine yet for hepatitis C, though researchers are working on it. Clinical trials of HPV vaccines are also in the works, with products expected to reach the market within the next five years. Researchers are testing potential HIV vaccines, though so far no one has hit pay dirt.

One other note on prevention for men: Circumcision lowers the risk of catching HIV. Men with a foreskin are eight times more likely to have HIV, and eight times more likely to give it to a partner, male or female.

After the Fact: Common Complaints

If you have skipped ahead to this chapter after having sex with a new partner, you may have gone searching on the Internet to determine the reason for that nagging sensation below the belt. The trouble with Internet sites is that many assume that you know what you have and are looking for more information. STD sites list every disease that survives in warm wet tissue without mentioning how common each is. They list "itchiness" or "bumps" as symptoms for a host of diseases—everything from herpes to gonorrhea to molluscum contagiosum. Good luck diagnosing yourself without seeing a lot of graphic and very scary photos.

So we are going to work backward, starting with a list of common complaints that may occur after sex, and what they mean. Some are STDs, some aren't. The STDs we'll be dealing with, in roughly descending order of likelihood, are HPV; herpes; chlamydia and gonorrhea; hepatitis B, A, and C; syphilis; and HIV. The non-STD conditions that sometimes mimic these diseases include yeast, bacterial, and urinary tract infections. We'll also throw in a discussion of pubic lice and pelvic inflammatory disease (PID), just for good measure.

Bumps or Sores on the Genitalia

Everyone's nether regions have a few bumps, but some warning signs should make you concerned. If a new bump is red and painful, or if it is oozing or wartlike, or if you find several new bumps at once, go see your doctor.

If a new bump is a symptom of a disease, the most likely culprit is the *human papilloma virus* (HPV), which causes genital warts. HPV is common. According to the Centers for Disease Control, "By age 50, at least 80 percent of women will have acquired genital HPV infection." It is also usually not a serious health risk.

You can get warts anywhere on your body, including the groin. About a week or two after sex, you may notice anything from subtle skin changes—a new area of dry scaly skin, a change in skin color, or an area raised from its surroundings—to textbook-clear warts. Or you may see nothing, because the warts are internal or otherwise difficult to notice.

There are a hundred strains of HPV, and where you develop the warts depends on where you came into contact with the virus, and what strain you're dealing with. Only about forty strains are sexually transmitted. When Samantha, a thirty-something patient of mine who was in a monogamous relationship, developed a bump the size of a pea on her right tonsil over the course of a month, she was understandably distraught. When her ear, nose, and throat doctor told her it was HPV she did the dreaded Internet search and became convinced that she'd gotten the virus from oral sex with her boyfriend, that her boyfriend was therefore cheating on her, and now she had genital warts in her throat. But after a long discussion with me about the differences in viruses and their transmission, she came to understand that the HPV strains that invade the genitalia aren't the same ones that cause throat warts. A little liquid nitrogen cleared up the problem, and a little more knowledge stopped her from peeking at her boyfriend's appointment book.

For guys, the warts that result from HPV aren't aesthetically pleasing, but there's no long-term damage. If the warts form in a noticeable or uncomfortable place, your doctor can burn them off with liquid nitrogen. This doesn't cure the virus—and you can still pass it to others—but it does solve the cosmetic problem.

For women, however, HPV is a different story. Of the forty strains that infect the genital tract, about thirteen can cause cervical cancer in women by entering the cervical cells and causing mutations in their genes. Often, these strains of HPV won't cause any visible warts, so you won't know you're infected until you have a Pap smear and get the results.

If you do get an atypical Pap result, though, I cannot stress enough that you should not panic. For starters, nearly every woman who is not a nun will develop an HPV infection at some point. If your Pap shows changes related to HPV, your gynecologist will likely tell you to come back in six months and have another Pap. About 80 percent of young women shake the virus on their own within one or two years, just as you would shake the common cold. If your immune system doesn't take care of the problem, your gynecologist can perform an in-office procedure to get rid of the offending cells. It takes a while for cervical cancer to develop, and if you and your doctor stay on top of an HPV infection, you can stop the disease in a precancerous phase. Pap smears aren't fun, but a yearly Pap is crucial to maintaining good health. If you're a sexually active woman, find a gynecologist as soon as you become sexually active (or when you turn eighteen if you're not sexually active yet) and visit her every year, or even twice a year if you have multiple partners. Plenty of cancers can't be prevented, but cervical cancer is one that can.

Other culprits for genital bumps and sores include the dreaded *herpes simplex virus.* Herpes is common, though your risk of catching it from any one encounter is low. The herpes virus is transmitted through direct skin contact. When the virus hits the skin, it finds its way to nerve endings at the skin surface, then winds its way toward the ganglion (the central cell that makes up the nerve), then spreads to neighboring nerves. Herpes tends to stay localized. HSV2, or "genital herpes" (what we're talking about in this chapter), stays in the genitals, and HSV1 or "oral herpes" hangs out around the mouth.

When you contract herpes, your first outbreak will occur about a week after contact. This initial outbreak will be more severe than any recurrence. It starts with a tingling or pain somewhere in the genital or anal area. Then comes fever, aches and pains, swollen lymph nodes around the genitals, followed by an outbreak of painful red spots that become blisters. These blisters then break and become ulcers. Over the next ten days, the ulcers crust over and heal, signaling the end of the outbreak.

At this point, the virus lingers in the nerves, but the immune system has kicked in and suppressed it. The suppression may last forever, or the outbreaks may come back from time to time. Stress, a decrease in immunity because of infection, a trauma to the genital area (rough sex, for instance), or even sunlight can trigger another outbreak. The average person with genital herpes experiences an outbreak once every three months, but these outbreaks can happen every few weeks, or never. It depends on your immune response.

Secondary outbreaks last for fewer days, lack the flu symptoms of the first occurrence, and produce fewer lesions. Treatment remains the same, with three choices of antiviral herpes drugs: Valtrex, Zovirax, and Famvir. Most doctors prescribe Valtrex because patients take it twice a day, versus five times for Zovirax and three times for Famvir. All work by slipping into the viral DNA and stopping replication.

People with herpes can manage their disease two ways (or three if you count doing nothing). You can wait for an outbreak, then take one to three days of treatment (ten for the first occurrence), or take the medicine daily to keep everything in check. Other than trying to reduce stresses that trigger new outbreaks, there's not much else to do, except avoid giving the disease to your partners. Herpes medications do lower your risk of spreading the disease, but they don't reduce the rate to zero. Side effects include nausea and headache, though few people stop taking their medicine for these reasons.

HSV1, which causes cold sores around the mouth, is much more common than HSV2. About 80 percent of us have been exposed to HSV1 at one time or another. Many of us don't even know we have it; we may just get cold sores when we're stressed or run down. The good news is that the immune response your body mounts to HSV1 translates into partial protection from catching genital herpes. So if you've ever had cold sores, you have a lower risk of contracting HSV2, and you may have fewer recurrences if you do catch it.

While you can catch genital herpes in the mouth, or oral herpes in the groin, this viral cross-pollination doesn't happen very often. These viruses like their own turf, and HSV1 infections that occur in the groin generally cause fewer and less severe outbreaks than those caused by HSV2.

Uncommon Sores

Other diseases that cause genital sores are rare. If you have one blister or ulcer that is red or oozing, and possibly painful, or just ugly, you might have developed the solitary lesions of *syphilis* or of *Hemophilus ducreyi* (*chancroid*).

Chancroid is more common in developing nations, so you should suspect the disease only if you recently had sex in, say, Africa, or had sex with someone else who just had sex in Africa. Chancroid lesions are painful but treatable with antibiotics.

Syphilis, too, is treatable with antibiotics, but if it isn't treated, it can come back in different forms over the next several years. The original ulcer, or chancre, is usually painless and will resolve after a few weeks. Then the infection goes into a latent, asymptomatic stage for one or two years. Secondary syphilis shows itself at this time with painful, scaly red spots on the palms and soles. These, too, will go away on their own. After that, the second latency period can last up to ten years. Unfortunately, when syphilis comes back for the third time, the microorganisms invade the brain, causing depression, dementia, and eventually death.

Fortunately, syphilis is treatable, as long as you seek medical help long before you ever get to the dementia/death phase. If you have a single painful or painless ulcer on the genitals, or multiple flat warts on the groin or around the rectum (another form of syphilitic infection), quickly schedule a visit to the doctor, because a shot of penicillin will stop the disease cold.

Although syphilis used to be widespread, it isn't common anymore in the United States except in the gay community (about 60 percent of infections are diagnosed in men who have sex with men). People with syphilis often turn out to have HIV as well. Since HIV needs to be diagnosed and treated as soon as possible, if you're a man who has sex with other men, syphilis symptoms should send you to the doctor right away. Most other folks with sores on their genitals, however, are far more likely to have a disease such as herpes than syphilis.

Testicle Pain

Sexually transmitted viruses and bacteria don't often travel to the testicles, so if your balls are sore after sex it's virtually guaranteed to be a mechanical issue. Infections take time to show symptoms. If your testicle pain occurs within a day or two of your encounter, and you don't have sores on the skin surface, you've likely just been bouncing around too much. Take some ibuprofen or Tylenol to dull the ache.

If the pain lasts more than a few days, go see a doctor to make sure you don't have some other non-STD guy problem. For instance, the epididymis, a small gland that wraps around the testicle, can get infected by the same varieties of bacteria that cause sinus or throat infections. In a few cases, gonorrhea and chlamydia (see below) can climb all the way up there. Alternately, your testicle may have twisted around the vessels that supply it, cutting off blood flow. If you are reading this chapter, though, this is not your problem. If it was, you'd be in too much pain to do anything other than go screaming to the emergency room, which is where you should be, since torsion of the testicles can preclude your ever needing to read the pregnancy chapter.

Irritation and Itching

If you're female, and it hurts to have sex, your genitals are terribly itchy, and you've got a discharge that smells or tastes like bread, only not as pleasant, you likely have a *yeast infection.*

These infections, caused by a fungus called *Candida albicans,* are as common as HPV. About 75 percent of women will develop a yeast infection at some point in their lives, usually after doing something that alters the acidity of the vagina. This can be anything from taking antibiotics to traveling, sitting in a wet swimsuit too long or having sex with a new partner, which is why yeast infections can look like STDs. Some infections feature an obvious white cheesy discharge and pain from the irritation, others are mild and just annoyingly itchy.

Yeast infections can be cleared up with over-the-counter creams or suppositories such as Monistat. However, if you've never had a yeast infection before, you should visit your doctor to make sure that's what you do have. If you do have a yeast infection, your doctor can prescribe Diflucan, which is a pill, not a suppository, and is more pleasant to deal with.

If you don't have a yeast infection, you'll need a different action plan to clear up the problem. If you have an STD, for instance, yeast infection medications won't help you. You might also have a bacterial infection and not a yeast infection. *Bacterial vaginosis* shares symptoms with yeast infections, including itchiness and a bad smell (though often more "fishy" than "yeasty"). Some bacterial infections are sexually transmitted, others result from douching or problematic underwear, but over 20 percent of women are affected whether they know it or not. Fungi and bacteria are different creatures; bacterial vaginosis will require antibiotics to clear up, as will *trichomoniasis,* a similar condition that causes itchiness and odors.

When it comes to vaginal infections, follow your nose. Any recurrent odor, especially if the odor is more noticeable during or after sex, deserves a look. Treatment for all of these bacterial infections is just a one-day course of antibiotics, so there's no harm in getting treated, and getting your partner treated as a precaution. About a third of male partners will have the same infection, and you want to be sure he doesn't give you the infection right back.

While most women have had or will have a yeast infection at some point, most men don't know they can get the same thing. Men's fungal infections are commonly called *jock itch,* and feature red, scaly, itchy skin in the groin. Over-the-counter jock itch spray clears the problem up, unless you're not circumcised, and the fungal infection has taken over the warm, moist area beneath the foreskin. Then jock itch starts looking a lot like women's yeast infections, with itchy, oozing, painful red skin and white discharge.

Yeast can also grow in other dark, personal places. One patient of mine, Max, kept coming into the office complaining of rectal itching. Usually, this turns out to be nothing more than a hygiene issue. You can clear it up by buying some medicated baby wipes at the grocery store and using them in addition to toilet paper. In a few days, the skin heals up and the itch goes away. In Max's case, however, the itch wouldn't stop for weeks. Max was a twenty-something hairstylist, and he was barely able to work without stealing away to the closet for some furious scratching every few minutes. Not only was this driving him crazy, his colleagues and clients were starting to notice the rhythmic ass-shaking during his styling sessions.

This gentleman was openly gay, and having sex with one committed partner without protection. Most of my gay patients are very safe and I was impressed that this couple, like many others, got tested before having unprotected sex and continued to get tested regularly. All my patient's STD tests came back negative, and swabs of the skin never showed any problem. Just as I was about to give up hope, he mentioned that his partner was having a problem as well. Sure enough, his partner had developed a yeast infection, and what my patient had was a case of rectal jock itch.

It doesn't matter where you put it, anyone with a yeast infection or jock itch can pass it to a partner. A one-day course of Diflucan for each of them cured the problem.

Itchiness Involving Small Creatures

Unlike the other organisms mentioned in this chapter, *pubic lice* are actually tiny insects that crawl around on your hair follicles, bite you, lay eggs, defecate, and then, exhausted from the effort, die. Usually you notice the itching first, then you look closely and see these little critters playing merrily on your genitals. If that doesn't provoke a panic attack, nothing will.

While nits are gross, they're rare–I've never seen a case in private practice–and they're a pure hygiene problem. Keep clean and keep clean partners. Your doctor can give you a topical treatment that will get rid of the bugs, and you can also use over-the-counter lice creams or shampoos. Then thoroughly wash your sheets and clean your clothes to avoid being reinfected.

Pain During Urination

Men and women can both get *urinary tract infections* when the bacteria kicking around the genitals enter the urinary tract, though the geography of women's personal regions makes them more susceptible than men. UTIs feature discomfort during urination, cloudy or bloody urine, frequent bathroom trips, and sometimes back pain and fever. While the "pain during urination" part mimics STDs such as gonorrhea and chlamydia, UTIs aren't STDs. Like all other bacterial infections, though, you'll need a prescription antibiotic to clear them up.

Women can limit their chances of getting UTIs by wiping from front to back after urination, urinating after sex, and keeping well hydrated. Cranberry juice inhibits the ability of bacteria to cling to the wall of the bladder, and thus can help you avoid UTIs as well.

Discharge in Men and Women

In general, any new gunk coming out of somewhere you've not seen it before should have you on the phone with your doctor. The most common cause of discharge is urethritis, or infection of the urethra.

Urethritis, according to one of my patients, feels like "pissing razor blades."

You'd think that a few razor blades in the urinary tract would move people to seek medical care immediately, but I've seen folks wait weeks. Why? They're scared to hear they have the most common causes of urethritis, namely, chlamydia and gonorrhea.

Chlamydia is a sexually transmitted parasite that can infect the urethra and epididymis in men, and the cervix, uterus, and fallopian tubes in women. Gonorrhea is a bacterium that does exactly the same thing. So most doctors treat you for both. About 5 percent of people are infected with some combination (one or both) of these diseases at any given time.

These infections are easily treatable with a dose of antibiotics that's not much higher than you'd take for a sinus infection, so there's no reason to avoid the doctor for fear of the cure. Your doctor, or the local walk-in clinic, sees these diseases all the time. No one is going to snicker while writing an antibiotic prescription. In fact, since it's only a one-day course of two 500-mg tablets of Zithromax and one 500-mg tablet of ciprofloxacin, you can likely get samples from your doctor to save you a trip to the pharmacy. Ask if he's got them on hand. Consider your diagnosis a learning experience, and be better about using condoms in the future (after talking with your partner– see "After the Diagnosis," below).

Actually, if you're female, you're lucky, in a way, if you show symptoms–most women with chlamydia are asymptomatic. Since roughly one of every twenty women reading this passage has the infection, you should be screened regularly. Ask your gynecologist to test you for chlamydia at your annual exam, or even every six months if you have a lot of partners. Getting treated can prevent pelvic inflammatory disease (see below) and infertility, not to mention spreading chlamydia to people who *will* have symptoms.

Abdominal Pain in Women

Many women experience cramps before and during their periods, but any serious, persistent lower abdominal pain is a potential problem, particularly if you are running a fever. These are symptoms of *pelvic inflammatory disease* (PID) and may be accompanied by vaginal discharge, pain during urination, and pain during and after sex. PID is caused by organisms–generally gonorrhea and chlamydia–that invade the genital tract, entering through the vagina and cervix, continuing into the uterus and fallopian tubes, and infecting all these stops along the way. Untreated, PID leads to serious health issues and can be fatal. Even when treated, PID can cause scarring, which can lead to infertility and tubal pregnancies. Tubal pregnancies are almost always fatal to the fetus, and can be fatal to mom. Bottom line: If you have any of these symptoms, have your gynecologist check you out. When in doubt, visit the doctor rather than hoping it will go away.

Irritation and Bleeding After Sex

If minor irritation or bleeding occurs right after you have sex, within the first twenty-four to forty-eight hours, then there are two possibilities. One is that you had an allergic reaction to your condom or lubricant. Allergies can cause skin reactions that look like poison ivy, or might be more subtle, such as minor redness, itchiness, and maybe some bleeding. Try switching condoms or lubricants and see what happens.

The second possibility is simple mechanical difficulties. With all the friction that goes on during sex, you can definitely cause soreness and some interesting cuts and bruises. One of my patients had a large sore right on the tip of his penis. We worried it might have been syphilis, but after a few questions, we realized that his new boyfriend had braces on the back of his teeth.

All bacterial and viral infections take time to enter the skin and replicate to the point of causing clinical symptoms. This latency period can last for weeks to months, but is rarely less than a week. Therefore, any symptoms that occur immediately after intercourse likely aren't STDs.

Feeling Ill

The more serious STDs cause massive reactions in your system when you're exposed to them. Herpes, the various strains of hepatitis, and HIV all cause flulike symptoms anywhere from one to six weeks after the encounter. Sometimes the flu is just the flu, but watch for these potentially worrisome symptoms:

> • **A faint rash, very swollen lymph nodes, and an extremely sore throat, often with visible ulcers.** HIV often manifests itself with these immune system–related symptoms.
>
> • **A change of color in the eyes, stool, or urine.** Hepatitis often causes these symptoms when it destroys liver cells, impairing the normal production and excretion of pigments in the bloodstream and intestinal tract.
>
> • **Fever and chills, accompanied by painful red bumps and swollen lymph nodes in the groin.** These are a dead giveaway for herpes.

Any of these symptoms are a major, flashing neon sign to call your doctor and figure out what's going on.

Postsex Action Plan

People who are sexually active should get in the habit of being tested for STDs at their annual physicals, or annual ob/gyn exams if that's your current source of primary health care. While the risk of catching a disease from any one encounter is low, the risks are cumulative, and sexually active people with multiple partners, or a series of partners, have a good chance of encountering some disease along the way. Getting tested and treated early saves you much trouble later on.

Most people, however, aren't in this habit. So if you've just had sex with someone you're not so sure about, or you didn't wear a condom, or it broke, you may be looking into testing for the first time.

Here are the details: Many tests on the market don't look for bacteria or viruses, but rather the antibodies to these bugs. After exposure, the body needs six or more weeks to mount a response that can be picked up on a screening test. So I'm in the habit of giving my patients who aren't being routinely tested this action plan for that postcoital moment when your head lands back on your shoulders and you realize you did . . . *what?*

1. Evaluate your partner's risk. Anyone could be infected, but common sense dictates that some people are riskier than others. Prostitutes, drug users, and promiscuous partners all put you at higher risk, because what are the chances that the young man you picked up at a party has never done this before? If you used a condom, on the other hand, with a friend-with-privileges you know doesn't sleep around, your risk is likely lower.

2. Get tested soon after your liaison. This test may or may not pick up anything you caught from the sex in question, but it can show what you had before. Not all STDs have obvious symptoms; for example, anyone can have an asymptomatic chlamydia infection kicking around for years. Now's a perfect chance to clear that up, and a baseline test can keep you from blaming a partner who's not at fault. Instead, you'll need to warn *him* or *her*.

3. Relax. You've got six weeks till your next test, so don't worry about it. There's literally nothing you can do. Turn to the section on stress relievers and anxiety if you're tossing and turning.

4. Six weeks later, go back for another test. If nothing comes back positive on the second test, then you're 99 percent clear. If you want to be sure, come back in about six months, at which point test results are just shy of 100 percent positive.

Facts About Testing

Gonorrhea and chlamydia are diagnosed by testing a swab from the affected region, or by testing a culture from a urine sample.

Blood tests can be used to diagnose HIV, hepatitis, syphilis, and herpes; in all these cases, we test for the antibody to the disease, not the disease itself.

The best way to diagnose herpes or syphilis, however, is not with the blood test (which only says that you've been exposed, not whether the current lesion is a result of that exposure). Rather, we swab the ulcer and see what caused it. For this, you need an active lesion, and the earlier you get it done, the better the sensitivity of the test.

Another reason you'll need an active lesion for a herpes test is that the antibody test is notorious for its high false positive rate in asymptomatic, low-risk individuals. If you have painful bumps and have had sex with people whose herpes status you don't know, a positive test is likely truly positive. But virgins have been known to get positive tests, too. For this reason, many doctors don't use the herpes blood test unless the patient has symptoms or has had recent risky contacts.

HPV is tough to test for, since there is no reliable blood test. HPV can be diagnosed through cervical biopsy in women after a Pap smear shows irregularities. External lesions can be tested by applying acetic acid to the suspect bump. If it turns white, you've got warts. This sounds like a do-it-yourself project, but trust me, you don't want to pour vinegar all over yourself every time you see a bump. Just go to the doctor.

After the Diagnosis

Some STDs run rampant through the population, and some viruses can sneak around condoms. Diseases can spread when neither party has symptoms, and they can lie latent for months or more. Sometimes STDs show such subtle symptoms that only a test can tell what you have. So it's difficult to pin down when you picked something up. This is especially important for couples to know. If a new bump appears, or the herpes test is positive, the first question everyone asks is "Who was cheating?" But the answer isn't as easy as the question.

Two married couples I've seen demonstrate the dilemma that a new STD can pose. Chris and Samantha had been married for ten years. During Chris's annual physical, I noticed a pimple on his groin, which he said reappeared every few months. Not only did it test positive for herpes but, after we delicately told Samantha, she tested negative. Somehow, Chris had had a case of herpes kicking around since a college fling, and had never known it. Even with a transmission rate close to 16 percent per year (for men to women; it's 4 percent for women to men), if you get lucky, you can go years without passing it along. Immune systems differ, so if one partner is diagnosed, that's not enough proof for a jury to convict for infidelity.

Of course, it can be fairly damning proof, too, if the person is guilty. Beth and Donny, the second couple, were both attractive, high-powered types, and had been together since they were teenagers. They had lost their virginity to each other. Alas, both men and women can wonder what's on the other side of the fence. At age forty-five, Beth decided to take advantage of all her business trips to see what she missed in college. Before one such trip, she came in with a few painful bumps. When the test results came back, I tracked her down in Europe to tell her that it was indeed herpes. She was expecting the worst, though, and was woman enough to tell her husband. Fortunately, Donny tested negative, just as Samantha from the first couple did. Now Beth is taking suppressive therapy, and Donny's still clear. Of course, dealing with the emotional trauma of infidelity isn't as easy as popping some pills. Donny and Beth were able to preserve their marriage, but only after months of counseling.

In the Interest of Full Disclosure

It's sobering to think that so many people are running around with herpes, chlamydia, and other diseases, but there's no doubt they are. Partly that's because these diseases are sneaky and get transmitted no matter what we do, partly it's because people are lazy about using condoms, but also, it's because there's a lot of denial surrounding these diagnoses. Most young professionals view getting an STD as a life-changing event. STDs are only supposed to happen to dirty, kinky perverts, not nice people like us.

Knowing that many people have the same disease softens the emotional impact of the diagnosis. Knowing that most STDs are treatable or resolve on their own should ease your fears. But after the diagnosis sinks in, it's time for the biggest challenge: notifying your partners. As much as it sucks to hear from your doctor that you've got herpes, it really sucks to have to call the people you've been intimate with and make this information public. It's largely because it sucks so much, and so few people do it, that these diseases are so common.

My recommendation to these timid souls is: *Suck it up, and do it anyway.* Yes, it sucks, but so does going to the dentist, and you do that. Be an adult about it and do your intimate friends a favor by saving them the uncertainty over what they might have picked up. You've suffered some embarrassment with your diagnosis, so now it's time to balance that with a strong dose of character and integrity.

Of course, you may be worrying what your partner will think of you now. If your partner was a one-night stand, who cares what he thinks? If you were or are close, then the same affection should move you to act in your partner's best interest. Regardless, any current partners need to be treated or they can give whatever you've got right back to you. While a chlamydia infection is bad, treating it and then getting it again two weeks later is even worse. I won't pretend making that phone call is easy. But it's necessary. It might help to look at the situation as one of my patients did.

Frank came in with a dramatic case of herpes after an episode of unprotected sex with another guy. I started him on treatment and at his follow-up visit a week later, his lesions were clearing. So we sat down to discuss what would happen next.

The first message, of course, was to wear a condom. The second message was that he needed to notify his partners. To my surprise, he'd already done so. Frank explained his philosophy. Everyone going into this game of sex, he said, is an informed adult. We all know that sex without condoms, or even sex at all, has risks. Getting an STD didn't make him a bad person. However, it was up to him to prevent the next case. So he made his round of calls, letting everyone from the past two to three months know the situation. Turns out, his partners weren't angry, but were thankful to know they should get checked. They appreciated his concern for their safety. Your partners will, too.

Part of what makes that telephone call so much tougher is that even though STDs are common, few people talk openly about them. So I recommend couples start talking about STDs early on. There's no need to discuss STDs and you. Just discuss STDs in general–research news you see, stories in the newspaper. Initiate a conversation about another couple's successful experience dealing with a disease. Start talking early, and eventually you can talk about yourselves. The goal is to take the secrecy out of STDs. If you expect your partner to fess up without prompting, or you put him or her on the spot, you'll miss an opportunity to become closer as a couple.

I certainly try to put this topic of conversation on the table when I think people are peddling disinformation and fear. At a fund-raiser, for instance, I walked past a klatch of women in the corner chatting about previous men in their lives. Hearing the word *herpes,* I introduced myself as a doctor and let them come back around to what they'd been talking about. One woman told me that she had been happy with her last suitor, but when he admitted he had herpes, she declined the next date. Did I think she made the right decision?

In a word, no. I gestured to the lineup of tuxedo-clad men at the bar. "See those guys?" I asked. "Out of those ten, probably two have herpes as well, and might not even know it." She was shocked. "This guy was open and honest enough to tell you," I said. "Open and honest guys are hard to come by. You could get to know him without having sex, and if you fall in love with him, you could take the necessary precautions." I told her how low the risk of transmission was when a couple uses condoms and the infected partner takes his medicine. "But if you go on a date with someone else," I continued, "there's a one in five chance he'll have it, too, and he might not be man enough to admit it, putting you at potentially even greater risk."

If a partner you're fond of does have an STD, remember, that doesn't make him or her a bad person. These are viruses and bacteria we're talking about, not someone's character. By separating people from their medical problems, STDs become the bugs they are, not a taboo to blush and stammer about.

Risk of Transmission

Now let's talk numbers. The Internet is wonderful for helping people learn more about their health, but one of the most frustrating things about it is that sites devoted to STDs tend not to tell you how common any given disease is. Spend some time at a clinic and you'll realize that if one out of every five patients has herpes, but you go weeks without seeing syphilis, chances are a patient with a genital sore has herpes, not syphilis.

If you are reading this chapter after a bout of unprotected sex, you want to know what your actual chance of catching a disease is. I can't give an exact number, but the following percentages are what we know to the best degree of certainty available.

If You've Had Sex, What's the Risk?

HPV. HPV is so common you almost certainly *will* be exposed at some point in your life. During any unprotected encounter, you have a 15 to 20 percent chance of being exposed and infected. Of course, this means that you've also got an 80 percent chance of not being infected. If you're worried, remember next time that condoms reduce the transmission rate by 70 percent.

Herpes. In monogamous couples where the man has herpes and the woman does not, her risk of catching the virus from him is around 16 percent per year. If she's the infected party, his risk is even lower—about 4 percent. This is without taking any precautions at all. No condoms, no drugs. So as you might guess, even though 22 percent of the population has herpes, the likelihood of catching HSV2 from a single encounter with a person of unknown infection status is low–well below one in a hundred. Condoms reduce the risk by about 60 percent, and if your partner is taking suppressive medications such as Valtrex, that drops your risk by half again. The virus is most active when lesions are present, so while you can still catch herpes when someone is asymptomatic, steering clear of any suspicious lesions is a great way to further limit your risk.

Chlamydia/gonorrhea. About 5 percent of the population has one or both of these diseases at any given time. If you have unprotected sex with an infected person, you're likely to catch these diseases yourself. However, condoms offer near complete protection. So do yourself a favor and turn that 5 percent chance into a less than 1 percent chance next time you have sex.

HIV. Here's a little secret they never told you in health class: At least in this country, HIV isn't very contagious. You have only about a one in four hundred chance of catching HIV from an *infected* person during a single act of unprotected sex. Since so few people are infected, your risk from any encounter with a person of unknown status is even lower. The risk is lowest for men having sex with women, higher for women having sex with men, and highest for men having sex with men. As a side note, women have lower levels of the virus during ovulation. However, since this gives you a rather large chance of getting pregnant, I wouldn't view ovulation timing as a good method of AIDS prevention. While that one person out of four hundred who has sex with an infected partner and catches HIV will feel unlucky indeed, the bottom line is that when it comes to HIV, the odds are in your favor.

Hepatitis B. Unfortunately, hepatitis B is about one hundred times more contagious than HIV, meaning that your risk of catching it from an infected partner is one in four. However, since most people who have hep B keep it in check with their immune systems, you only need to worry about the people with chronic infections. Not counting people in the first stages of disease, 0.5 percent of people in the United States have the virus and can transmit it, which gives you about a one in a thousand chance of catching hep B on any specific encounter.

Hepatitis C. Don't worry about this one unless you've had direct blood contact. Even then, the risk of transmission from an infected person is only around 3 percent. Since 1 percent of the population is infected and contagious, this puts your risk at around .03 percent per exposure to blood of any kind.

Things That Raise Your Risk

The above numbers, reassuring as they may be, are just averages. Some activities raise your risk. For instance, STDs are more prevalent in some parts of the world than others. Generally, when people say a region is a good place to get laid–say, Thailand–steer clear. I've got several patients who came in at the end of their holiday trip to Brazil. Three out of four brought back something from their vacation–one case of chlamydia and two cases of herpes. Yet somehow, the one guy who didn't catch anything has already rounded up some other friends to go back next year.

Aside from location, the more body fluids you are exposed to, the higher your risk. If a person has open sores, for instance, then bacteria and viruses can enter the bloodstream through the equivalent of an open door. This explains why people with one STD are at higher risk of catching and passing on another. Menstrual blood can also pass along pathogens, meaning women are more contagious at that time of the month.

Also, sexual activities that result in abrasions or bleeding can raise your risks quite a bit. For most people, this means anal sex, which can involve a great deal of trauma and microscopic tears in the skin. Any STDs that take root in the genitals can be transmitted to the anal area, and these microscopic tears offer a perfect entry point for diseases to enter the bloodstream–much better than the mouth. We don't see many cases of genital herpes, HPV, or syphilis in the throat from oral sex, but these show up all the time in people's rear ends. They often progress to later stages there, too, before people seek treatment. This is partly because neither you nor your partner looks into this area, and because anal itching and pain can occur from normal conditions, like hemorrhoids. If you've been on the receiving end of anal sex, and are experiencing discomfort, then ask your doctor to shine a bright light there and take a look. In general, vaginal sex is safer than anal sex, and oral sex is safer than either. Condoms are safer than no condoms, and sex with anyone sporting an open sore or lesion is a big "no."

Low-Risk Activities

One of my patients struck me as quite the family man, but his one vice was his habit of ending up at a massage parlor after a late night at the office. We're not talking a platonic rubdown at a spa here, but one that has a higher price tag for a few fringe benefits.

So after a few happy-ending massages, he came into my office because the thought burrowed into his brain that he might catch something from the masseuse's hand job and pass it along to his wife. But he didn't need to worry, as the tests confirmed. It's quite difficult to catch anything from a hand job. STD bugs don't last long on nongenital skin, so manual sex is nearly as low on the risk list for transmitting diseases as holding hands. That said, the risk isn't zero. These viruses do have *some* life expectancy on surfaces, so any repeated intimate contact can transmit disease. But of all the things with sex that can get you into trouble, hand jobs should be low on your list of worries. I wish my patient would have worried more about shoring up his relationship with his wife.

Likewise, you're probably not going to go far enough with exotic dancers or strippers to catch anything–unless you're paying top dollar. If you go into a private room and have to negotiate a price for a specific act, best to be cautious and get tested.

A Note About HIV

Even though HIV is rare in the United States and the risk of catching it from any encounter is low, people have a lot of questions about the disease, so it merits its own section. First the good news. This scariest of STDs is becoming more and more manageable in the United States. Life expectancies are rising, and death rates have fallen since the first antiretroviral drugs came on the market. While AIDS has devastated Africa, most people here who are diagnosed with HIV can expect to live relatively long, full lives. Even people who aren't diagnosed until they develop an AIDS-related illness have very encouraging odds.

That's the good news. The bad news is that HIV is a difficult disease, requiring complicated drug regimens to control. Some of these drugs have nasty side effects, including fatigue, nausea, diarrhea, fat loss in certain areas and gain in others, rashes, and long-term cardiovascular problems.

One of the toughest parts of the disease, though, is the stigma that still exists about HIV. Because of this, many people are reluctant to go to a doctor to be tested. Several home HIV tests have come onto the market for precisely this reason.

In general, these tests are as good a first screen for HIV as what your doctor can do. However, unlike home pregnancy tests, I'd advise against taking HIV screening into your own hands. The benefits of having professional counseling outweigh any concerns you might have over who finds out or what happens next.

For example, if the test is negative, who cares if your doctor sees it? Getting tested for HIV is a prudent part of health maintenance, and doesn't imply anything about your habits.

But if the test is positive, you're not going to want to be by yourself. You're going to want to get counseling, get set up with a good HIV treatment center in your area, and you are going to want your insurance company to pick up the tab. Your doctor can help you swing into action on these things. She can't if she doesn't receive the news with you. HIV is a serious diagnosis, but being alone to receive it is even worse.

The Healthy Guide to Avoiding STDs

There are plenty of sexually transmitted diseases floating around that do nefarious things to your body, but the fear and misinformation surrounding these diseases are just as bad. I've seen people avoid treatment for weeks because they're too scared or ashamed to hear a positive diagnosis. The takeaway from this chapter is that while you should certainly try to avoid catching STDs, many are truly no big deal to diagnose and treat. If you don't get bent out of shape about a sinus infection, you can deal with chlamydia or gonorrhea. If you contract herpes, you can keep it in check with medications and avoid passing it to your partners by using condoms and abstaining during outbreaks. HPV won't give you cervical cancer if you have regular Pap smears. Even HIV is no longer a death sentence. So if you're concerned, get tested. Not knowing will keep you up at night more than knowing and making a plan with your doctor for treatment.

The best way to avoid those late-night worries is to keep your STD risk as low as possible. Limit your partners—anyway, sex is better with a long-term partner who knows what turns you on. Wait to have sex until you get to know your partner and can discuss STDs. Use a condom unless you're in a monogamous relationship and both of you have tested clean. Sure, unprotected sex with a stranger may get your adrenaline racing, but before you dive in, think how you'll feel when your heart is racing as you wait to hear a test result. Sex is supposed to be fun. STDs make sex not fun. You owe it to yourself, your partners, and your health to have the best, most worry-free sex possible.

Seven

Drugs and Drug Testing

NOT TOO LONG AGO, a friend of mine, Tom, called to tell me he was trying to leave his hedge fund job for an analyst position at a research firm. It was a move he'd wanted to make for a long time, so I was happy to hear it. He'd wowed his interviewers, and was negotiating a package that would make the new gig quite lucrative.

As soon as Tom officially got the job, though, his new company asked him to go to a clinic for preemployment drug screening. That's when he panicked.

Now, this man did not fit the stereotype of a drug user. Tom was earning a generous six-figure salary at one job, then landed an even more generous paycheck at the next place. If you asked him about the fundamentals of any company in the industry he researched, he could reel them off without glancing at his notes.

He had, however, gone on a major cocaine spree at his birthday party a week before he got the drug clinic appointment. He came into my office with visions of his entire career dissipating like a cocaine high because of one wild night.

I calmed him down, took blood and urine samples, and showed him a little something two days later: Both tests came up negative.

Tom was surprised, but if he'd done a little research into this field alongside the companies he covered, he wouldn't have been. Cocaine, like many illicit drugs (with the notable exception of marijuana), is water soluble. Because your kidneys process the water in your body quickly, cocaine and its metabolites are detectable for around two or three days in the urine. After that, they're not. So I advised him to take his drug test with confidence–but also to take his panic as an opportunity to rethink his drug use. After all, he might not have so much warning the next time, and there's plenty of other reasons to quit as well.

Like most young adults, my friend grew up sitting through DARE classes (Drug Abuse Resistance Education) and listening to ads telling us to "Just say no." Like most young adults, he didn't listen. Well over half of eighteen- to twenty-five-year-olds have tried an illegal drug at some point. Add in the nine million Americans who use prescription drugs for "nonmedical reasons" as the National Institute for Drug Abuse puts it, and you have a lot of people getting high, stoned, or tripping. Whether we like it or not, drug use is a rite of passage in high school or college, and there's no indication that this is going to change any time soon.

Certainly, as far as unhealthy living goes, illegal drugs are as bad for you as anything else in this book. Certain drugs–for example, crack and heroin–are incredibly addictive and lead to serious health problems after minimal usage. Use any drug daily, including marijuana or cocaine, and you run a much greater chance of your occasional indiscretion turning into a self-destructive habit. I don't know anyone with a daily drug habit who doesn't suffer significant health effects. Drug use also has a high correlation with stupid behavior. Stupid behavior can lead to a trip to the hospital or morgue if you're not careful, because suicide, homicide, and accidents are all more likely when you're intoxicated–whether you're high on pot, cocaine, or booze.

But with all the drug hysteria you see on TV or learn in school, real information gets lost in the screaming. I'm confident that when people get straight, sober information on drugs, they'll choose not to use them, and encourage their friends and loved ones to do the same. I also want to make sure that ambitious young people don't miss out on great career opportunities because they think last month's Ecstasy hit will show up on a drug test. I want to let employers know the limitations of the tests they rely on to keep the workplace drug-free.

It's important to keep in mind when reading this chapter that the drugs listed here are completely illegal. Whether you agree with the war on drugs or are lobbying to legalize marijuana, the reality is that possession of many of these drugs can land you in jail, and jail is certainly bad for your health. Even if you don't end up incarcerated, I've seen many careers nipped in the bud when people get caught in drug tests, get raided at parties, or become too drugged to function. Your best bet to avoid trouble with drugs is to avoid taking them.

But since at least half of young people have chosen not to avoid drugs even though they're illegal and unhealthy, I'm writing this chapter to answer the questions I've been asked by patients over the years. Telling a young person that something is illegal rarely deters them. Tell the same young person that a drug can give them a hole in the brain or make them shake like someone with Parkinson's disease, and they think differently. Use the information below to make an educated choice not to do drugs, and you'll be a step ahead of the game.

Marijuana

Marijuana is the most popular illegal drug out there, so we'll look at that first.

In order for any drug to have an effect on your body, it must bind on a molecular level to specific receptors. The THC in marijuana smoke binds to receptors in the areas of the brain that are responsible for short-term memory and motor coordination–specifically the basal ganglia, hippocampus, and cerebellum. When THC binds to these receptors, you experience short-term amnesia and bouts of clumsiness. In short, you get stoned.

Unlike other drugs, though, marijuana doesn't bind to many other areas of the brain beyond these three. Your brain's core functions–regulating breathing, heartbeat, and blood pressure–take place in the closely guarded brainstem. While many "downers" bind to receptors in this critical brain area, marijuana does not. No matter how much you smoke, your lungs and heart will keep plodding along as usual. For this reason, it's virtually impossible to die of a pot overdose. You might die if you do something stupid like driving while stoned, but it won't be an overdose that kills you.

All sorts of people try marijuana—one government study found nearly 54 percent of eighteen- to twenty-five-year-olds had tried it. But most people don't try it all that much. The same study found that only 6 percent of the teen and adult population had smoked marijuana in the past month. If you assume that these percentages don't change much over the years, then it stands to reason that there's well over a hundred million people in this country who have smoked pot, including a couple presidents in recent memory, but nowhere near this many people let marijuana become a habit.

Despite the ads claiming that pot is a gateway drug, it turns out most people try marijuana, find it interesting, but not that exciting, and return to their basically drug-free lives. Some people continue to use the drug on occasion as a way to relax, but outside of college, few people smoke so much pot that it would affect their health. While it is true that most crack addicts have tried marijuana, most pot smokers will never try crack.

Like smoking cigarettes, smoking lots of marijuana can lead to pulmonary disease. There are about eight times more tar and pollutants in a joint than in a cigarette, so chronic pot smoking gives users a greater risk of cancer or emphysema than cigarette smokers. Add in the memory loss and motor coordination trouble pot causes in the short run, and it should be clear that pot certainly isn't good for you. The damage is not necessarily permanent; as noted in chapter 2, if you're young, your lungs have a remarkable ability to heal themselves from the damage you inflict. If you only smoke pot on occasion, the effects of your last joint will fade within twelve hours. If you smoke daily, you'll need closer to thirty days to return to normal.

"Thirty days" is a key time frame with pot, because marijuana can also take a month to leave your fat cells. THC is lipid soluble, meaning that unlike most illegal drugs, THC is stored in fat, not water. If you smoke pot regularly, THC seeps into your fat cells, then slowly leaches back into the bloodstream, where it's excreted by the kidneys. Since your body sheds the contents of fat cells a lot more slowly than it sheds water, you can test positive for THC up to a month after you last used pot. This can be a problem if you need to take a random drug test (see the testing section, below).

While there aren't any good studies on how marijuana affects your health in the long term, it's safe to say the biggest dangers come more from the way pot affects your judgment than how it affects your body. Today's marijuana will get you baked. The pot your parents smoked in the 1960s had about 3 percent THC. Thanks to the miracle of selective breeding, pot now has 6 to 13 percent THC.

The high level of tar and pollutants in marijuana does worry some people, so I'm often asked whether some ways of ingesting or inhaling marijuana are safer than others.

While the best way to avoid marijuana's pollutants is to avoid marijuana, eating the drug causes less harm than smoking it does. Lung tissue is extremely sensitive, and the tar and carcinogens in marijuana smoke are toxic. The stomach, on the other hand, is a much tougher organ, since its job is to break down anything you eat into its most basic components. The stomach is well-protected from carcinogens, and the substances that are toxic to the lungs in marijuana smoke are harmless to the stomach when the plant is ingested.

The only caveat to this is that many pot smokers crave the rapid high that smoking gives. The blood vessels in your lungs have about the same surface area as a tennis court. One puff of smoke into the lungs gives you maximum exposure to THC, which goes directly into the bloodstream and on to the brain. Your stomach isn't nearly so efficient: The plant must be broken down by stomach acid, then the THC must come into contact with the intestinal wall, and then be processed by the liver before it continues its journey to the brain. You'll absorb the same amount of THC whether you eat your pot or smoke it, but with eating, you might not get high for an hour. Not all pot smokers are willing to wait that long, but if you are, you'll have a much healthier set of lungs (if not a waistline) in the long run.

The second least damaging way to use marijuana is to smoke it in a water pipe. The small number of medical studies out there on water pipes shows that pipes and bongs make excellent filters. Many of the studies focus on the use of the large water pipes (or hookahs) popular in the Middle East for smoking flavored tobacco, but other smaller studies have looked specifically at marijuana smoke.

The water in a bong offers two advantages. First, it acts as a filter, removing tar and other pollutants from the smoke. Second, the water cools the smoke, so you're less likely to burn your airway. Unfortunately for those intent on getting high, the same water that is filtering the toxins from the smoke also does an effective job of trapping THC. This means that many people will smoke more, and more deeply, from a water pipe than from a joint in order to get the same high. This offsets some of the benefits, though not enough to cancel them out.

Smoking a joint or pipe is the least healthy way of getting that pot buzz. Unlike a cigarette, there's no filter between you and the pollutants in a hand-rolled joint. And also unlike a cigarette, there's no insulation. You inhale very hot smoke, which is likely to burn your throat (just as the joint can burn your fingers if you're not careful). This, plus the high amount of tar and other chemicals in pot, leads to the hacking coughs that people who smoke frequently experience. The thermal damage to the upper airways is compounded over time, and can lead to scarring and breathing problems.

Like any drug that causes a high, marijuana can impair your judgment. So if you're getting baked, you should take care not to put yourself in dangerous situations. Don't drive. Make sure you have a way home, and get someone to take a break from stoning to act as a chaperone and make sure you avoid any stupid behavior.

The biggest danger I see with marijuana is the tendency for people to self-medicate with it, often masking more serious issues that require medical help. Depression is a big one; marijuana relaxes you and lets you forget your troubles for a while. But pot is a very inefficient way to treat depression. Daily use brings all sorts of side effects that antidepressant medications don't even begin to approach.

One young patient of mine, Caitlin, had been struggling for years with the loss of a close relative. She would barely make it through work each day, then she'd come home, have dinner alone, and smoke until she passed out. For over a year, she had no boyfriend, no friends, no vacation; just marijuana and her job. I don't know whether the depression or marijuana came first, but they were linked by the time Caitlin and I talked.

I could see right away that any antidepressants I could prescribe, or any lifestyle changes she tried to make, would be thwarted by her reliance on pot. It's tough to break out of chronic pot smoking, because the escape from reality and the calming effect of the drug really do make tough times seem easier. Unless someone can break through your pot haze and show you that the drug is keeping you from improving your life, you won't be motivated to quit.

So Caitlin and I spent a lot of time looking at the various issues she was dealing with. She knew she had become antisocial, and she didn't like that, but she didn't see what she could do about it. With a few conversations, I was able to convince her that her pot smoking was actually her way of treating the classic symptoms of depression. But unlike antidepressants, which would help her get better, marijuana was just providing an escape from her misery and robbing her of the motivation to change.

She agreed to give my advice a try, and cut her smoking down to once or twice a week. She started taking Wellbutrin for her depression, and began seeing a therapist. A few months later, she was back to dating again and was spending more time out with friends and colleagues than at home alone with her bong. I doubt Caitlin would have had this kind of recovery if she hadn't changed her smoking habit.

Marijuana can also mask bipolar disorder. I once treated a teenager, Gina, who had a history of erratic behavior and smoking pot. Every time Gina came into the office, she reeked so badly of marijuana that I was surprised everyone in the waiting room wasn't getting high as well. She would alternate between skipping school to smoke pot and running away from home for weeks at a time. Her mother had once called me because the girl had taken her brand-new car to a Brooklyn chop shop and sold it for about half of what it was worth. Gina blew through the cash by the end of the week, then showed up stoned to crash on her mother's couch.

Sure, Gina had a drug problem, but again, the drug use was both a symptom of her personality disorder and a way of self-medicating. Without marijuana to smooth her manic episodes and provide an escape from the lows of depression, her bipolar disorder would have been even more damaging. It took several months and many different medications, but with the right changes she was able to get effective treatment for the bipolar disorder and escape her reliance on marijuana.

I have also seen a number of patients trying to treat their anxiety disorders with pot. June worked as a counselor in a cancer center. The patients loved her because she was so empathetic, but that empathy made it tough for her to stop thinking about her patients' troubles when she went home. After working at the center for a few months, June developed a sore throat. Rather than do what most people do for a sore throat (suck on a few lozenges) June became convinced she had developed throat cancer. This made her so distraught that she wound up with terrible insomnia and stopped seeing friends or dating in preparation for what she viewed as her imminent death.

When June came in to see me, she spent her first few appointments announcing that she was going to die. Since a quick check of her throat revealed no real problems, I calmed her down and asked her to talk about her fears for a while. It turned out that she had been smoking marijuana every day for years, until she stopped one day because she had that sore throat. On further questioning, I learned that she'd had a long history of anxiety dating back many years; however, once she started her daily smoking, the anxiety became much more manageable. Basically, she had been treating her anxiety disorder with daily doses of marijuana, and as soon as she stopped, the very sore throat that had prompted her sobriety became the source of a full-blown panic attack. Marijuana had allowed her to distance herself from reality.

June was pretty tough to treat. It took weeks of therapy and a combination of antianxiety drugs to get her back on an even keel.

But finally, with the right medications, she was able to feel as good as marijuana had made her feel without marijuana's bad side effects.

If you are smoking pot frequently, and find that you need it to be functional, emotionally stable, or even detached enough to get through life, then talk with a doctor or psychiatrist and ask them to evaluate your emotional health. Your doctor can help you find therapies and drugs for both depression and anxiety that are more effective, legal, and better for your lungs and your psyche than pot. While the lung damage and clumsiness pot causes are no fun, living in a haze because you can't deal with life is even worse.

Prescription Drug Abuse

Any drug can be abused, even if it was prescribed by a doctor and you buy it from a pharmacist, not a dealer. Seemingly normal people who don't look like addicts can still go to great lengths to get their fix.

Once, when I was working at a clinic in New Jersey, a nice-looking gentleman came in three times in a week for persistent pain. The answers he gave to all my questions pointed to a textbook case of kidney stones. Typical treatment for this condition includes pain control and hydration. He took a prescription for Vicodin, but then came back a few days later for a prescription for the stronger Percocet when he claimed the pain didn't subside. Then he came back a few days later saying he'd lost the prescription. By the time he called and said he was planning a three-week trip to Florida to care for his ailing father, and needed a longer prescription, it was clear something was up.

Sure enough, the pharmacy where he'd been filling his prescriptions told us he'd given that line to six different doctors in the area, and had attempted to fill no less than twenty prescriptions for painkillers. He had memorized the symptoms of a disease that required prescription-strength painkillers, and put his acting skills to use. He even spiked his urine sample with a drop of his own blood for good measure. Had he not frequented the same pharmacy, he could have kept this up all year.

Like the gentleman from New Jersey, many prescription drug

abusers favor narcotics such as Vicodin, Percocet, codeine, and Oxy-Contin. Doctors usually prescribe narcotics, derivatives of the opium poppy, to treat pain. Opium is the base that gives us morphine and heroin (in its most potent form). Folks get hooked on narcotics because in addition to pain relief, these drugs trigger opioid receptors in the brain that give users a sense of euphoria and well-being. Oxy-Contin, when crushed and snorted, can even give users a heroin-like high.

Unfortunately, opioid receptors, unlike marijuana receptors, are located in the brainstem. Too many narcotic painkillers can cause respiratory depression and death. Combine them with alcohol, which can also cause respiratory depression and death at high doses, and you get a compounded effect. A little alcohol and a few pills, relatively benign when ingested separately, can be lethal when taken together.

While narcotics are popular, they're not the only prescription drugs people abuse. Valium, Xanax, and other benzodiazepines are used to treat anxiety disorders and insomnia. They're excellent drugs for treating these conditions, but if you have an addictive personality, it's easy to become hooked on the calming effect. At that point, you become less interested in using these drugs as a bridge until you can make lifestyle changes, and more interested in taking these drugs to maintain your mood.

The trouble with diagnosing and treating prescription drug abuse is that all these drugs—unlike, say, heroin—have legitimate uses. People recovering from surgery need narcotics for treatment. Valium helps folks with anxiety disorders calm their nerves. So how does a doctor distinguish between those who truly need painkillers or tranquilizers, and those just looking for a high? A few warning signs can help you tell if your prescription drug use has turned into a problem:

You run out of drugs before you are supposed to: If I write a prescription for a week's worth of painkillers, the prescription should last a week. When someone comes back three days later for another round, I wonder where the extra pills are going.

You "lose" prescriptions: Nobody loses prescriptions for antibiotics or skin creams, but when it comes to painkillers, people become complete klutzes. I've had patients come back two hours later because their purses were stolen, they left their prescriptions on the bus, or they just can't remember where they put them. I keep waiting for someone to come in and say his dog ate his prescription.

You're "allergic" to less potent painkillers: This one is a classic. No one is ever allergic to the stronger ones, but I've heard a thousand times how someone is "allergic" to nonnarcotic painkillers, and even to weaker ones like Vicodin. In most cases, the ingredients are the same, but the dose is different, making allergies highly unlikely. If you're "allergic" to Vicodin, but can take stronger drugs without a problem, it may be time to get help.

You have a detailed knowledge of narcotic choices and strong preferences for what you'd like: Most patients who need painkillers are new to these drugs, or have only been on one or two in the past. While I'm all in favor of people taking charge of their health, I don't expect my patients to know the difference between Darvocet and Dilaudid, except in the most severe pain-management cases. When they do, I wonder why they have such an interest in doing their homework. Usually it's because they're hooked—and then I know we need to have an entirely different conversation than one about pain.

Drugs You Likely Won't Try

Few people who fit the health-book-buying demographic also fit the demographic of those who use drugs such as heroin and crack. But in case you're curious, here are a few reasons these drugs cause problems for those who try them.

Heroin and crack both cause rapid highs followed by equally rapid crashes. The crash drives the user to get the drug back into his system for a second immediate high. This cycle makes it very, very easy to become addicted to heroin and crack in a way drugs with slower highs and more gentle downs can't match. For this reason, you rarely hear about recreational heroin or crack users. Even someone without an addictive personality can get swept into junkie status after the first up-and-down cycle.

Heroin is extremely dangerous, causing far more emergency

room visits than its low rate of use (less than 2 percent of teens and adults have ever tried it) would suggest. Heroin can constrict airways, cause fluid to build up in the lungs, and destroy lung tissue. Injections of heroin can contaminate the bloodstream with bacteria, leading to heart valve infections or stroke. Dirty needles also give viruses a direct shot into your body, which is why heroin users often pass HIV, hepatitis B, and hepatitis C to other users.

Like heroin, crack cocaine has a reputation for destroying users' lives. Crack is much like cocaine except it's cheaper, usually smoked, and produces a more intense though shorter high. Like cocaine, crack can cause heart attacks, but since you smoke it, you add lung damage into the mix. Because the high is so quick and so short lived (as short as ten minutes), and because the crash is so unpleasant and crack is so cheap, people take another hit almost immediately. A few hits later, you need crack to feel normal. That's why newspapers, at the height of the 1980s crack epidemic, were filled with stories about people selling their TVs and furniture to buy crack.

You don't want to wind up that desperate. Best to steer far clear of both these drugs.

Party Drugs

Unlike crack and heroin, you stand a good chance of being around Ecstasy, cocaine, or crystal meth at a party sometime. All have highs that are attractive to late-night partyers, though all have side effects and risks that are a lot less entertaining.

Ecstasy

"E" is one of the most popular party drugs around, because it makes you feel euphoric, and everyone likes to be happy. While antidepressants such as Prozac make you feel happier over time by building up levels of serotonin in the brain, Ecstasy both slows serotonin's metabolism and causes your brain to release loads of this chemical instantaneously. So taking Ecstasy feels somewhat like taking three months of Prozac at once (this is merely an analogy; please don't try this at home).

Ecstasy is a social drug in the true sense of the word. Rats given the drug in isolation act less "ecstatic," so to speak, than those given Ecstasy in groups. By enhancing sensory perception, alertness, and well-being, Ecstasy makes social interactions much more intimate. You become friends with everyone at the party. You love the world.

Ecstasy first came on the scene in the early 1930s as a weight-loss drug. Then it enjoyed a brief renaissance in psychiatric offices when psychiatrists used the drug to enhance therapy sessions with patients. In theory, Ecstasy was supposed to make these patients more open and self-aware. Not surprisingly, Ecstasy turned out to make psychiatrists more aware, too, when—according to lore—they started using the drug themselves. In 1985, after determining that the drug had significant abuse potential and no legitimate medical uses, the U.S. government classified Ecstasy as Schedule 1, making it illegal to purchase or prescribe.

Ecstasy, like cocaine and other stimulants, causes your nerve cells to release dopamine and norepinephrine. This makes you feel alert and energetic, but also gets your heart racing, just as adrenaline would. When you're on Ecstasy, your blood pressure rises, your heart rate increases, and your muscle fibers contract. This contraction causes the "bruxism," or teeth-grinding, that most ravers experience. Just check out how many people at after-hours clubs are sucking lollipops or chewing gum.

A typical tab of E has anywhere from 50 to 150 mg of MDMA, Ecstasy's active ingredient, though most hover closer to 50 (that's dealer logic—why sell one tab with 150 mg when you can sell three with 50 mg each). Your body processes Ecstasy via a pathway that is easily saturated. This means that while your body can handle one tab over several hours, extra tabs increase the burden dramatically. Doubling your Ecstasy dose can quadruple the MDMA level in your blood. High doses create high levels of adrenaline. This increases your heart rate, raises your blood pressure, and constricts the small arteries that bring blood to your organs.

MDMA also raises what your body considers a normal temperature, causing hyperthermia (overheating), which can result in seizures and muscle breakdown. Overheating makes you thirsty. In extreme cases—if you drink the liters of water that ravers sometimes do—you can dilute your bloodstream to the point where your blood no longer supplies your cells with the electrolytes they need to function. This condition, hyponatremia, can cause seizures, or even death.

I won't pretend Ecstasy causes *a lot* of deaths. The annual death rate among Ecstasy users in a 1996 United Kingdom study was estimated at 0.2 to 5.3 per 10,000 users (heroin, in comparison, kills 81.5 of 10,000 users annually; automobiles 1 in 10,000). While there have been reports of deaths from small amounts of Ecstasy, most deaths are related to higher doses—five or more tabs at a time. If you're doing fewer tabs than that, you've got a very low chance of dying from the ingestion.

Just because you're likely to survive the habit, though, doesn't mean there aren't other factors to consider. For instance, there's the "hole in the brain" issue. Positron-emission tomography (PET) scans show the metabolic activity of cells in the body. PET scans of Ecstasy users reveal areas where neurons in the brain cease functioning after repeated use. These pleasure centers have released so much serotonin that eventually the cells give up. Fried neurons cause memory impairment, an inability to reason, and depression.

These changes are proportional to the amount of drug taken and the length of abuse, and are inversely proportional to the time since the last dose. Even occasional users will feel the effects of dopamine and serotonin depletion for a few days afterward. Take a hit of Ecstasy on Saturday and you may feel tired, depressed, and dull until halfway through the week. Memory loss and mood problems can last up to two weeks after the last dose. In heavy users, these effects may be permanent.

So there's depression and memory loss to consider. And then there's the depletion of the dopaminergic neurons that Ecstasy causes. The loss of dopamine-containing nerves leads to a condition that resembles Parkinson's disease—think tremors, rigid muscles, and frequent falls. This condition is permanent and unresponsive to treatment.

So here's the verdict on Ecstasy: A few tabs will affect your mood, motor function, and sensory perception for a few days.

Chronic use, especially heavy use, can lead to irreparable brain damage that screws up your personality and your ability to sit still without shaking. There is a small risk of dying from an overdose, though you can lower your risk by taking a few precautions.

Many people get into trouble with Ecstasy because they don't understand the immediate effects on the body, and how to combat these effects. Since Ecstasy raises your body temperature and dehydrates the body, staying cool and well hydrated is important. Unfortunately, this is easier said than done in a nightclub. Going outside the club every so often to cool down is a good place to start. Drinking a lot of water also cools the body, but ravers can go overboard and drink so much they dilute their bloodstreams, as described above. Drinks containing sugar and electrolytes (such as Gatorade or juice) can mitigate the risk of bloodstream dilution. But don't go for Red Bull or other energy drinks. These beverages increase the stimulant effects of Ecstasy and lead to dehydration, putting you at increased risk of side effects.

If you're at a party and you see an Ecstasy user becoming intoxicated—passing out, for instance, or moving uncontrollably or showing a lot of abnormal behavior—make sure that person heads to the hospital immediately. While there's no way to treat an overdose (the emergency room team will just monitor the person's body temperature and give him fluids), cardiac side effects are best experienced in a hospital. This is a rule to follow with all drugs: Seek help sooner rather than later. Sure, the hospital will "catch" the user with drugs in his system, but better to catch them there than at the autopsy.

Given the medical troubles Ecstasy can cause, I advise my patients who tell me they're using it to find safer ways to party. Other things can make you feel happy—friends, good music, sex, exercise, positive feedback at work, antidepressants if you're depressed—without causing brain damage.

Cocaine

Cocaine is derived from *Erythroxylon coca*, a shrub indigenous to South America. Like many other drugs, cocaine has legitimate medical uses. When applied directly to tissues, it causes blood vessels to close up and tissues to go numb. This is exactly what you need when doing surgery—numb tissue that doesn't bleed much. While other medications have the same effect without abuse potential, cocaine is still used by dentists and oral surgeons to provide local anesthesia before procedures.

When snorted, cocaine is absorbed into the bloodstream and goes directly to the brain, causing the release of epinephrine, norepinephrine, dopamine, and serotonin. All stimulants work on these same neurotransmitters (chemicals that transfer information between your brain's neurons). It's just the ratio in which these chemicals are released that determines the effects of different drugs. Ecstasy, for instance, primarily affects serotonin and therefore sensation and mood. Crystal meth, through its increase in epinephrine and norepinephrine, makes you more aware and better able to concentrate. Cocaine has some elements of both of these, making you feel alert and euphoric.

While these neurotransmitters make you feel high, it's what cocaine does to the rest of your body that causes harm. Cocaine increases your heart rate and constricts your veins. Constricted veins mean higher blood pressure. You can experience two blood pressure peaks with cocaine—one thirty minutes after your hit when drug levels in your system are highest, and one about ninety minutes later, when the drug's metabolites (produced as your body breaks down the cocaine) peak.

For most people, this increase feels like mild exercise: twenty to thirty extra heartbeats a minute and a ten- to twenty-point increase in blood pressure. But a few folks get unlucky and experience a far greater spike. It is possible to have a heart attack a few hours after taking cocaine. The risk is higher in people with clogged arteries or other heart disease.

According to national statistics, about 3.7 million people used cocaine in the past year, and about 175,000 of them ended up in the emergency room. Some 40 percent of these people complain of chest pain, and 6 percent of those actually have a heart attack.

This is a lot lower than newspaper articles and public health warnings about cocaine would lead you to believe. The reason for the disparity between actual heart attacks and the warnings about cocaine use is that every doctor has worked in an emergency room as part of her residency or rotations. Every doctor has seen a young, healthy adult, brought in by ambulance after a cocaine binge, wind up tethered to a respirator in cardiac arrest. Who in their right mind would trade a whole life for a thirty-minute high? Even if a drug has a relatively low risk of fatal side effects, those side effects still happen to someone. Enough bad things can happen in life already without sticking your neck out for more.

Studies have shown that many of cocaine's harmful effects are dose-dependent. This means that the more you do, the more problems you have. Sure, accidents and general stupidity can occur from one hit, but it's the folks who use a lot of cocaine who get into the most trouble. Most professionals and students value their functionality enough to use cocaine rarely, or maybe just once or twice in a lifetime.

If you do use cocaine, here are a few safety issues you should keep in mind. In addition to the cardiovascular risks, doing cocaine gives you a small—but real—risk of catching a disease. Everyone knows that sharing needles can spread HIV and hepatitis. What's less well known is that snorting cocaine or crystal meth carries the same risks. These drugs constrict all your blood vessels, especially the ones in your nose. This damage to your nasal membranes gives you a high risk of nosebleeds or even microscopic bleeding you can't see. When you use the same straw or rolled-up dollar bill as the guy before you, small bits of blood from his nose can mingle with the blood in yours. Viruses don't need much encouragement to make the leap. The risk is lower than if you're sharing needles, but it is a risk, and a preventable one. So if you're not going to say no to cocaine, at the very least don't share your straw.

Also, since higher doses of cocaine cause more trouble than lower doses, moderation is key. If you are going out, leave the drugs at home, or at least parcel out a very small amount, rather than your whole stash. The last thing you need at four in the morning is several grams of coke in your pocket waiting to be snorted. When it's done it's done. If you're truly craving more coke (an addiction warning sign if you are) your lack of coke in hand might be enough to make you go home.

And home is where you should be, because you should never go shopping for drugs while you're banged up. If you've burned through your stash, that's bad enough, but once you go on the prowl for more, you not only increase your risk of a drug overdose, you also put yourself in physical danger. Drug dealers aren't known for being nice guys. It's best to avoid them in general, but even more so when your brain's not fully functional.

Like all drug users, those who use cocaine are playing Russian roulette. Even if you don't normally have an addictive personality, you may get hooked on the high and dislike the crash so much you go for the next hit. It's fairly easy to slip toward dependency and the kind of serious consequences that land you in an emergency room. You don't want to be that statistic every doctor remembers. You won't be if you drop the habit.

Crystal Meth

Like cocaine and Ecstasy, crystal methamphetamine is a stimulant. It's a little-known fact that the Vicks company (the folks who make the nasal sprays and chest rubs) originally used crystal meth as a nasal decongestant, but it proved too potent for frequent use. By changing the molecule slightly, the company was able to make a much less powerful drug that could still unblock your nose. Without another pharmaceutical usage, methamphetamine made its way to the black market.

Since crystal meth targets slightly different chemicals in your brain than cocaine or Ecstasy, it produces less of a euphoric effect. Instead, crystal meth makes you awake, alert, and full of energy. Ravers will use crystal meth to keep going another hour, while truck drivers like this drug for its ability to keep them awake on long hauls.

So what's the downside? Same as the others: The rush of adrenaline drives up your blood pressure and heart rate. This puts you at risk for heart attacks or other cardiac damage. When crystal meth is snorted with friends, it can be contaminated with viruses including

HIV or hepatitis B and C. If you're looking to stay awake, better to have a double espresso instead of trying this drug.

Other Party Drugs

At a really raging party, unfortunately, you stand a chance of taking a party drug you didn't mean to take.

One such drug is Rohypnol, a sedative that's similar to Valium, Klonopin, and Xanax. The main difference is that "roofies" start acting quickly, and are quite potent. Even a small dose causes an immediate loss of inhibitions and memory.

Anesthesiologists use Rohypnol to prepare patients for surgery. Rapists use it to prepare women for sex. Not only do roofies relieve inhibitions in the intended victim, they make the victim forget anything that happens after the dose. While you may want to forget what's going on with, say, a colonoscopy, you do want to stay functional at a party where your safety's at risk.

GHB is another common date-rape drug. Scientifically known as gamma hydroxybutyrate, this drug was originally introduced in the late 1980s as a bodybuilding supplement. GHB targets the GABA receptors in the brain, just as alcohol and Valium do. The drug causes sedation at higher doses and increases libido, euphoria, suggestibility, passivity, and amnesia, all of which make victims easy targets for sexual assault. When slipped in a drink, GHB can make your cocktail taste salty or soapy, although flavorful drinks will cover that up.

To avoid accidentally taking Rohypnol or GHB, stick to clear drinks such as vodka or gin, so you know if something tastes funny. Take your drinks straight from the bartender or mix them yourself. If someone you don't know or don't trust insists on buying you a drink, go to the bar with him. Always party with friends who will look out for you, and if you suspect something is amiss, have a friend escort you home as soon as possible.

Determining the "Safest" Drugs

I'm often asked which drugs are safest to use. While all are illegal, and none are truly safe, some are likely to do less harm than others.

One such manufactured drug is ketamine, an anesthetic. This drug makes you feel separate from your body, as though you were floating away through a "k-hole," as users call it. Because ketamine is difficult to make in a basement, most of the illegal supply comes from legitimate sources such as veterinary or doctors' offices that have failed to keep an eye on their stocks. Because the supply comes from doctors' offices, ketamine is less likely to be adulterated, poisoned, or diluted than other drugs. Users obtain the sealed pharmaceutical vials, then bake the drug down to snort the residue.

Ketamine is very safe to use during surgery. Whether the average drug user is as careful as an anesthesiologist is debatable. What is clear is that ketamine does not cause vasoconstriction, and so is less likely to damage the nasal mucosa than cocaine. The only toxic side effect is a remote possibility of respiratory depression (and hence death if you're not treated). I've been searching through the medical journals for a documented case of death from ketamine alone, and I've yet to find one. This is not to say that it can't happen, but you'd have to try pretty hard to die using it. Just do me a favor and don't try so hard.

Drug Testing

Like my buddy Tom, who came in panicked about his recent cocaine binge, many of my patients work themselves into a lather over their employers' drug-testing policies. Plenty of companies have started testing new hires, though many of the baby-boomer executives at these companies don't have a clean history themselves. One woman I know was being recruited to work at a company by a manager who, at a social function, told her that he'd actually been arrested for selling drugs back in the day. Then he invited her to smoke pot with him (she declined). The next week he e-mailed her to say, sheepishly, that the company had instituted a drug-testing policy.

I have also spoken to many HR execs and entrepreneurs who want to know if drug testing will help them ensure a drug-free workplace. These folks want to know which tests are the most cost-effective and efficient so they can pick new hires who won't let drugs hamper their performance.

Urine testing is the most common way of testing for drugs in the workplace. These tests are popular because they are cheap and effective. The standard protocol is to test at hiring and rarely, if ever, thereafter. Those industries that need sober employees to protect the public interest do random workplace testing (think military and airlines), but this is rare in most of the private sector.

One obvious limitation of testing new hires is that you won't catch all drug users. These planned screenings involve a time delay between scheduling and the actual appointment. This delay can be several days or weeks. The only people such screenings will catch are:

1. Those not smart enough to stop
2. Those too addicted to take a week off
3. Marijuana users who get stoned so often that the THC has saturated their fat cells

Occasional users can definitely slip through the cracks. As an employer, you likely won't find out about an occasional drug user's habit until his performance starts to slip. Random drug testing might catch such a person, but not necessarily. If you test during the week, a weekend drug user can easily have all the drugs out of his system by Tuesday.

If you do decide to use urine testing, the most sensitive test uses a mass spectrometer, which looks at the weight of the molecules that pass through it. Every molecule has a specific weight based on the number and type of atoms that compose it. Mass spectrometry is tough to beat. Molecules are what they are.

Many companies, however, save money by ordering dipstick testing rather than the more expensive and sensitive mass spectrometer. Dipstick tests are more easily fooled by the many adulterants reported in chat rooms online, though the testing companies do try to stay abreast of the latest adulterants out there. If a dipstick test reports the presence of these adulterants, it raises a red flag.

People also try to beat dipstick tests by drinking copious amounts of water or using diuretics (including goldenseal, a medicinal plant popularly used as an adulterant) to dilute their urine. This makes particles less concentrated and harder to detect. Of course, testing centers know this, too, so a urine sample will be rejected if it's too dilute. This means the person will have to retake the test later.

False Positives

While most drug testing questions I hear are from drug users hoping to beat these tests, some nonusers worry that other substances will cross-react with a drug test and cause false positive results. All drugs have to come from somewhere, and many have harmless relatives derived from the same source. Poppy seeds, for instance, can make a drug test come back positive, because poppy seeds contain various amounts of morphine and codeine. But poppy seeds only cause positive test results within twenty-four to thirty-six hours of ingestion, and the ratio of morphine to codeine in poppy seeds is well known. Urine samples that differ from this ratio will be taken as evidence of narcotic abuse, not evidence of a poppy seed bagel.

If you don't use pot, but do like hemp products, you should know that many of these products, from candies to extracts, can cause positive tests. This is tougher to get out of than the poppy seed positive, because legally, THC is treated as THC, and your positive test will stand despite your plea that all you did was eat a hemp sandwich. If there's drug testing in your future, leave the hemp at home.

Amphetamines can show up in your system from a variety of legitimate sources. The most common are decongestants (pseudoephedrine, phenylpropanolamine), ephedrine, and diet pills (phentermine) including some from Mexico (Asenlix, Fenproporex). Drug tests can usually differentiate between methamphetamines and amphetamines based on the orientation of the molecule and the ratio of methamphetamine to amphetamine. Last night's Ecstasy hit will not be mistaken for cold medicine. But the Mexican diet pills, which contain methamphetamine, might trigger a positive Ecstasy test. Keep this in mind if you are shopping for diet pills online.

Another little factoid: Vicks nasal spray can also trigger a positive Ecstasy test. Vicks contains L-methamphetamine, while Ecstasy contains D-methamphetamine, which is almost identical but over ten times more potent. Fortunately, most testing centers do a confirmatory test looking at the specific orientation of the molecule to differentiate the two, so it is unlikely that treating your nasal congestion will give you a positive test.

Nothing is going to trick the machine into a positive test for cocaine, benzodiazepines (tranquilizers like Valium or Xanax), or barbiturates. However, all these drugs have legitimate medical uses, so if you have a prescription or have had oral surgery or dental work recently, make sure you have documentation before going in for testing.

Before many positive tests are ruled on, the supervising physician may contact the subject to see if there is a legitimate medical reason to have a positive test. This involves asking about any documented use of the above substances as well as looking for signs of drug abuse. Only after these inquiries will the test be considered "positive." Policies differ among employers, but be prepared to answer any questions if they arise.

Timing

The easiest way to beat a drug test is to not do drugs. But if you've done drugs in the past and are clean now, I want to assure you that a few indiscretions will not kill your chances of getting a good job. Since most drugs are water soluble, your kidneys process them and excrete them quickly. For example, almost any dose of heroin is completely excreted in less than twenty-four hours. For most other drugs, even heavy use will have cleared the system within three days of quitting. Occasional users can test negative within a day.

The only exceptions to this are PCP, barbiturates, and marijuana. I'll skip over the first two, since they're not that popular, unless you live in 1960. Marijuana, on the other hand, wins drug popularity contests hands down.

THC is fat soluble, with levels building up in fat cells over time. If you smoke one joint, your body will filter out the THC over a day or two. Smoke more, and THC levels in your fat cells rise. This means that after you stop smoking, the THC will leak out of your fat into the bloodstream for days to weeks. A daily smoker needs up to thirty days to test clean. There's no fixed rule for people in the middle, so figure that the more you smoke, the longer you'll be in the danger zone.

While many people try to get around this physiological fact, you can't change your fat cells as quickly as you can turn over the water in your body. There's no way to change your physique substantially (losing big chunks of your fat) in a few days or weeks. Even if you took all the crash dieting suggestions in the diet chapter of this book, a 160-pound person with 20 percent body fat might lose 10 pounds in two to three weeks. Even if all 10 pounds were fat, you'd still have 22 pounds of fat left, and they will still shed THC despite your best efforts to the contrary. So while working out is always a great idea, when it comes to passing a drug test, you won't be helping matters.

Hair Testing

Drug testing can be performed on virtually any body tissue, and while blood and urine remain the most popular options, hair testing is a possibility. Certainly, many of my patients worry about hair testing, with good reason. A four-inch piece of hair has been on your head for ten months. Longer hair may have been around for years. So while most drugs leave your system in a few days (or a month, with pot), your hair could, in theory, reveal your bong habit from college.

Your hair is made up of an inner cortex and an outer cuticle that protects the cortex. Toxins are deposited in the inner cortex in proportion to their levels in the bloodstream. Most drugs, including marijuana, crystal meth, cocaine, opiates, and LSD can be detected in the hair.

Hair tests are best for detecting chronic drug use, because only tiny amounts of drugs can be deposited in the tiny cortex of the hair over a few days of occasional use. If you used cocaine at a birthday party six months ago, and have been clean since, a hair test likely won't show your onetime use. On the other hand, a daily habit will cause a positive test, even if you quit a few months ago.

In my experience, employers rarely test hair because it's time consuming, expensive (ten times more expensive than a urine test), and doesn't address the problems most companies are concerned with. Most companies drug test not because they care whether people smoked pot in college, but because they want to make sure the people they hire won't skip work, embezzle funds to pay for a drug habit, crash their cars into coworkers in the parking lot, or blow major deals because they're too high to care. A simple urine test is a cheap way to answer this question, so that's the test most employers choose.

Of course, some companies spring for hair testing. One man I know was given a hair test because he was a crewman on a yacht, and the company wanted to make sure that those piloting its 150-foot vessel had been and would be clean. You sometimes see hair testing in divorce or custody hearings, wrongful firing trials, parole or criminal hearings, or lawsuits. But unless you give someone a compelling reason to suspect drug use, or you are going for a position of great responsibility such as law enforcement, health care, or a few executive positions, you are unlikely to have your hair plucked for testing.

I've heard people give all sorts of reasons for failing a hair test, but the most common is the claim that the drug on the sample came from the environment. On first glance, this seems plausible–our heads are out in the open every day, while our urine and blood are not. If a neighbor has a crack habit, in theory, trace amounts might show up in your hair.

But folks who go to the expense of hair testing are wiser than that. Labs wash the hair repeatedly and test the washings for drugs. When the washings are drug free, the labs digest the hair with enzymes and test to see what drugs are locked inside the cortex. These interior substances definitely came from your bloodstream, so "Someone dropped LSD on my head" is not going to fly.

On the other hand, the testing labs do admit that some of the things we do to our hair can obscure positive results. Bleach, peroxide, and lice shampoo, for instance, can mask marijuana in your hair. Peroxide might cover up Ecstasy or methamphetamines, and perms or straightening chemicals can obscure results for a cocaine or opiate test. All these can cause negative or obscure results when the person is not negative.

But if you don't do drugs, you don't need to worry about anything cross-reacting and giving you a false positive hair test. No matter how many poppy seed bagels you enjoy, the only thing that will cause you to fail a hair test is an illegal drug habit.

When to Get Help

Drug tests have their limitations, but if you're at the point where you're bleaching your hair to mask your pot habit, it's time to step back and look at the situation. When recreational drug use turns to abuse or true addiction, you need to see a doctor or visit a drug treatment center to learn how to quit and get your life back on track.

Recreational drug users, by definition, can quit at any time. When I've seen people who fall into this category, I recommend they stop—it's better for your health in the long run—but I realize that people also need to know how to recognize if their habits are creeping toward abuse or addiction.

Drug use becomes drug abuse when things start going wrong, and you keep using drugs anyway. A marijuana smoker who develops a chronic cough but keeps smoking is a drug abuser. Someone who skips work because he's withdrawing from a cocaine hit but takes another hit to ease the transition is a drug abuser. So, incidentally, is anyone who needs a shot of whiskey to get out of bed. It's not the use of a particular drug that indicates abuse, it's the person's behavior.

Drug abusers can still stop when they want to, but they'll have a tougher time of it than occasional users. A drug abuser doesn't really, physically crave his drug, he just has a continued desire for it despite feeling some of the side effects. A nudge in the right direction can still encourage the drug abuser to cut down or quit.

Once drug cravings set in, however, abuse becomes addiction. Addicts have an overwhelming desire for their drugs that supersedes reason and overpowers all other needs. The addict will skip work; leave relationships with friends, lovers, or family; and will lie or steal to get his drugs.

While some drugs such as crack or heroin have high rates of addiction, most recreational users of pot, cocaine, Ecstasy, and other drugs never approach addict status. But it's always something to watch out for. You can become addicted to *any* habit-forming drug, including drugs you can buy legitimately at the pharmacy. My patient who was hooked on painkillers, for instance, lied to doctor after doctor in the hope of getting his fix.

If your drug use is interfering with your work, your personal life, or your relationships, or even if it's just making you feel bad about yourself, it's time to put real effort into quitting, either on your own or with professional help. Start by asking your doctor what you can do. She'll likely be thrilled to help you, and can recommend counselors or programs. Depending on how hooked you are, she may recommend a combination of medical and psychological assistance, either in an outpatient or inpatient setting (i.e., rehab). When in doubt, ask for help. If you can't make that first phone call yourself, ask a friend to do it for you. The worst thing that you can do is nothing.

Eight

When You See Your Doctor

NO ONE ENJOYS BEING SICK, but from the fear you see in some people's eyes when you mention visiting a doctor, you'd think doctors still used leeches.

Whether it's because of an unexplained itch, a hacking cough, or an anxiety disorder, we'll all wind up in the clutches of America's medical system someday. And thanks to the miracle of modern medicine, you're likely to leave feeling better than when you came in. But that doesn't make going to the doctor any more pleasurable than when you were five and knew you'd be getting a shot. First you cool your heels in a drab waiting room filled with little but 1998 *Redbook*s, then you wait some more in an exam room while wearing an uncomfortable paper gown. Maybe your physician is someone you've known for years, but maybe you're new in town and this is the first time you're seeing her. You're not sure what questions you should ask. Maybe you'd like to tell her that you're so stressed at work you can't sleep, and because you can't sleep, you're becoming even more stressed at work. Maybe you've been drinking too much and would like to cut back, but you're worried what she'll think. Or maybe you've got a rash on your tush, but you're mortally embarrassed to bring it up.

In this chapter, I'll give you some tips for making the most of your encounters with the medical profession, including how to find a good doctor, how to pay, and who can see your medical records. But before I do that, I want to assure you that the most important thing you can do at the doctor's office is to bring up anything that matters to you.

For starters, you may have an actual problem, in which case the worst thing you can do is avoid treatment until something relatively benign becomes serious due to lack of care. Chlamydia, for instance, can lead to pelvic inflammatory disease (PID) in women if it's not treated. Or you may have something truly serious that only seems benign. I've seen people come in with heartburn that turned out to be heart disease, and swollen glands that turned out to be cancer. Asking questions about something that concerns you, no matter how small or silly it may seem, isn't neurotic, it's smart.

But even if your concerns turn out to be nothing, your doctor has definitely heard sillier things before, probably right before you walked in. I recently saw one well-connected lady who came in, put her bejeweled lapdog on the exam table, and told me she had a very serious case of fungus. She did not have a rash, mind you, but her friend, a hairdresser, had diagnosed said fungal infection over coffee. This woman was so sure about what she had that she wouldn't even describe her symptoms to me. Instead, she insisted I treat her with the strongest antifungal medicines I had. Since strong antifungal medicines have a host of potential unpleasant side effects, I wasn't about to write a prescription just to humor her. But she wouldn't listen to my explanations, and left, presumably to find a doctor who was easier to manipulate.

No sooner had she left than a young man came in and told me he had a testicular parasite. That was a new one to me. I've heard of parasites going many places in the body, but I'd certainly not seen one in the testicles before, and I couldn't imagine what one would be doing there anyway. But my young patient couldn't sleep because he was plagued with visions of worms crawling through his nether regions. A quick exam revealed that there was indeed a raised lumpy structure on his testicles–right where the lumpy structure known as the epididymis should be. A few reassurances banished those worms back to the imaginary land they'd come from.

So if you come in after folks like those and ask why your butt itches, your doctor will take a look and tell you—end of story. No laughing, no pointing. See, that wasn't so bad, was it?

How to Find a Doctor

The worst time to search for a doctor is when you desperately need one. So if you're reading this book and don't have a primary care physician, *now* would be a good time to start looking. (Uninsured? You can still look for a doctor. I'll address the insurance issue below.)

Women often choose to make a gynecologist their primary care physician in order to combine an annual Pap smear/pelvic exam with a more comprehensive physical. That's fine, but if there is more to you than a uterus and ovaries you're better off finding an internist or family practitioner as well. He or she will provide you with a thorough head-to-toe exam and a discussion of issues that don't involve your feminine side. Think of your ob/gyn as an extension of your primary care experience, not a replacement for it.

If you are insured and looking for a doctor, start with your insurer's list of doctors in your area, since you'll want to make sure your insurance company picks up as much of the tab as possible. You can ask your friends (or coworkers, since they share your plan) for recommendations. Your insurance company may even have feedback on in-network doctors; there's no harm in asking. Or you can leaf through the list and start making calls to ask the important questions:

> • **How long is the wait for a new patient visit?** Some offices only take appointments for new patients during certain slots, either because there's a lot of paperwork for new people to fill out, or because they like to make returning patients feel special by getting them in more quickly. Either way, you want to know that you'll be able to get an appointment fairly soon if you need one.

- **Does the doctor give same-day appointments?** This is important, because you don't want to be brushed off when problems come up. Even if you only see an associate or a nurse-practitioner, make sure that the office will accommodate you when you need to be seen.

- **How old is the doctor, and how long has she been in practice?** No, I'm not advocating ageism—you should ask this question so you can find the doctor you're most comfortable with. Younger doctors may be more up to date on current medical progress, but they're also less experienced. Older physicians are more experienced, but if their practices are nearly full, they might have less time for you. Go with what feels best. In general, the more time that a physician spends in an academic center—that is, a hospital connected with a medical school and a residency training program—the more likely it is that he or she keeps up with current treatment guidelines. Doctors who work at these centers are asked to train students and residents, and therefore need to stay on top of their fields.

- **Is she board certified in internal medicine or family practice?** You definitely want a doctor who is board certified in her area of practice, since that guarantees that she's finished a U.S.-accredited training program. Anyone with a medical degree and one year of internship training can practice medicine, and there are no restrictions on the scope of that practice. For example, if I wanted to hang a shingle and start doing boob jobs, there's no law that says I can't do it. For this reason, it's important to ask about the boards.

By far the most important question to ask is how well the doctor is going to serve your needs. Is she competent? Capable? Interested in hearing about your problems? Then you have a good doctor.

Some questions are less important:

> • What medical school did she go to?
> • Is the hospital that she's associated with the absolute best hospital in town?
> • Is she on the Best Doctors list?

Good medical schools can crank out mediocre doctors, and places you've never heard of can churn out competent, empathetic ones. You will want to evaluate your doctor's hospital affiliation if it looks like you will be spending some time within the hospital walls (for a surgical procedure, or birthing, for example), but I would still say that your choice of doctor is much more important. Check the hospital rankings, and their score on their latest review by the Joint Commission on Accreditation of Healthcare Organizations (JCAHO), which monitors hospital safety and competency, but don't dump a good doctor because the other hospital in town scored three points higher.

Doctor rankings also mean little. I've dealt with one office that was rated consistently near the top of *New York* magazine's Best Doctors in New York list. I was appalled by the service and care. Thanks to a great PR team, though, the office stayed at the top of the charts. If the Best Doctor ranking is the result of a peer survey—doctors rating doctors—it means a lot more, but many magazines, alas, don't bother doing their research.

What About Specialists?

It doesn't do you any good to have the world's foremost expert on the left kidney in your town if (a) you can't get an appointment and (b) you don't know what you have anyway. Unless you've got a long-standing issue, such as seeing a dermatologist for acne, or you have a chronic condition such as diabetes, few young people need a specialist on call. HMOs make people go through a primary care physician to see a specialist for a reason: Family practitioners see the whole litany of complaints, so they're less likely to jump to conclusions (hunting for an ulcer, say, because their specialty is ulcers, when the person is in fact having a heart attack).

If something ever does go wrong, you can start picking great specialists after the initial diagnosis. But even here, having a good primary care doctor on your side will make this stressful process that much easier.

What About Health Insurance?

Health insurance is massively expensive and bureaucratic. That's fine if you work for a large corporation that both offers insurance and can help you navigate the paperwork. But many young people work for small companies, or take temporary jobs, or work for themselves, or spend time between jobs, and don't have health insurance. Uninsured people often avoid preventive care, thinking doctors will charge exorbitant fees. Uninsured people also wind up in dire straits if they do have medical emergencies. There's nothing like a sudden case of appendicitis to wipe out your savings.

There are two things you should realize. First, you can usually purchase your own health insurance if you don't have an employer that offers it, and second, you can pay cash for medical services if you're uninsured. If you're up-front with the doctors and hospitals providing your care about your uninsured status, you can likely negotiate very good discounts. Neither solution is perfect—individual insurance can cost a bundle, as can paying out-of-pocket for anything beyond routine visits—but both are better than ignoring your health. This point is worth repeating: **If you are seriously ill, or worry you might be, get treated first and worry about paying for it later.** In a worst-case scenario, many doctors and hospitals will work out a payment plan with you.

If you decide you want to buy health insurance, visit a site such as www.ehealthinsurance.com for quotes. Search out any professional organizations you might join; some, such as the Freelancers Union, offer group health insurance rates in certain areas. Costs vary widely by state and type. Laws about coverage also vary widely by state (see the preexisting condition section, below).

If you're young and healthy, and your state allows it, your best option is a *catastrophic plan*. For a few hundred dollars a year, you can get a $500 to $1,000 deductible, although the price is usually higher in metropolitan areas. You'll cover your own doctor visits and basic emergency costs, but the insurance company takes care of anything over that. If you buy such a plan, put aside $50 to $100 a month for doctors' visits and deductibles. That way you'll never be caught off-guard.

If you can't find a catastrophic plan in your area, you may have to buy a basic HMO plan. Rates can run from $200 to $500 per month, even more for families. If you find a plan with lower premiums but various limitations on what kinds of care you can receive, that's okay. All health plans cover some portion of office visits, hospital procedures, and usually prescriptions. In order to offer you lower premiums, though, a plan might limit which doctors you can see, and make you responsible for a larger portion of the bill (a 20 percent copay, for instance, instead of $20). These limitations make life a bit more complicated at times, but you'll still get the care you need if you become ill.

Given how expensive health insurance can be, I'm not surprised that some young people choose to roll the dice and stay uninsured. After all, if you have an accident or become violently ill, you can go to an emergency room and they can't turn you away. That doesn't mean they'll take care of you forever, but they will fix you up well enough to put you back on the street. Then they will send you a bill for an exorbitant amount of money. If you're destitute, of course, you'll just add the bill to the pile.

If you're not destitute, but you're still not able to afford the cheapest health plan in your area, then you should put money aside every month toward health care bills. If you put aside $50 a month–the cost of a few pizzas and lattes–that's $600 a year reserved for doctor visits and, yes, you can use cash to pay for an office visit. Cash works the same way in a doctor's office as it does everywhere else. Simply tell the office this is how you plan to pay when you call. In fact, if you want, you can haggle over your doctor's fees as though you're buying a used car. Prices are set by the doctor or office manager, so don't take no for an answer until you've spoken with one of them.

If you come across as someone who pays when you visit, never bounces checks, and returns to the office, you may get a better deal than insurance companies do. Figure about $50 to $150 for a visit and $100 for lab work, depending on the tests. I've seen higher bills, but rarely more than a couple hundred dollars per visit. If you have concerns, you can always ask to have the minimum number of tests run, and ask for a quote from the lab beforehand. Doctors order tests in groups, or "panels," most of the time, but can often pare down the list by excluding irrelevant items from the panel. For example, you might just need certain liver tests, and not a complete metabolic panel. After you ask the doctor to order only the essential tests, take a minute to call the lab (most tests are shipped offsite to a central lab such as Quest, LabOne, or LabCorps) and ask for a quote. This should ease your mind about what you are getting yourself into.

A few hundred dollars for office visits and tests is a lot of cash, but primary care can help keep you out of the emergency room. That's where the bills really *do* stack up.

Preexisting Conditions

Nothing causes headaches like reading health insurance policy provisions on excluded "preexisting conditions." One reason people avoid being tested for diseases such as AIDS is that they worry a positive diagnosis, and hence a "preexisting condition" will raise their premiums or prevent them from obtaining health insurance in the future.

There is some good news about preexisting conditions. If you know you will be accepted for a new policy (for instance, your new employer covers all employees), then your new insurer will pick up the tab if you meet a few conditions. First, you must have had coverage similar to the policy for at least twelve months, with no more than a sixty-day lapse in between policies (this varies slightly between policies, but is fairly standard). If you meet this standard, your illness will be covered. So the number one rule for folks with chronic conditions such as diabetes is **don't let your insurance lapse.** Federal law allows you to keep your health insurance for up to eighteen months after losing a job, as long as you pay whatever your company was paying for insurance (plus a small administrative fee). This program is called COBRA, and it's worth looking into if you find you'll have time between jobs. Since your employer is responsible for making you aware of COBRA and helping you enroll, make sure you have this conversation before you actually leave your job.

In some states, such as New York, if you don't fall in this category—for instance, if you haven't been insured for a while—your new group policy will still eventually cover your preexisting condition; however, it generally won't pay for treatment for the first twelve months. But this isn't the end of the world either. If you have any sort of chronic condition, or just want to be prudent, follow my earlier suggestion to put away $50 or more a month to pay for treatment. If you let your insurance lapse for some reason, your medical savings can help with payments until your new policy kicks in twelve months later.

If you're obtaining insurance through your employer, your eligibility and premiums won't be affected by preexisting conditions. This means that if you're diagnosed with, say, AIDS, high blood pressure, or chronic back pain while you've got a policy, your premiums can't be increased. If you're starting a new job, and your employer offers health insurance to other employees who do the same job you do, then they have to offer it to you.

That's the good news. Unfortunately, there is plenty of bad news about health insurance and preexisting conditions, too. Many employers don't offer health insurance, and many young people don't have employers. If you try to purchase health insurance on your own, you can run into both very expensive policies and a maze of state laws. Some states allow insurance companies to reject you, if you're applying as an individual, for just about any reason—including a preexisting condition. Or the company can decline to pay for coverage for that condition for as long as you have the policy. If you are self-employed, or cannot obtain health insurance through your employer, it pays to consult a health care lawyer, consumer advocate, or insurance broker to figure out state laws and your options.

Urgent Care

Because doctors' offices are occasionally slow about granting appointments, and because many common complaints don't require a full history and physical, an industry of urgent care clinics has sprung up in most cities, and even in the occasional Target store.

If you don't have a primary care physician, these clinics are a great option. If all you've got is a simple urinary tract infection, back sprain, or ear infection, you'll get excellent care at a place that values getting you in and getting you out, and is *much* cheaper than the emergency room. All that matters is whether you can trust the doctor on call to identify anything that's more serious than it appears. For that, you're no worse off trusting an urgent care doctor than trusting any other doctor you don't know. Just check the diplomas on the wall, or ask the secretary about your doctor's board certification.

On the other hand, urgent care centers are not the best places to seek care if you have chronic conditions such as diabetes or high blood pressure. Many doctors have overlapping or even contradictory views on how to manage chronic conditions. For example, there are dozens of painkillers you can take for back pain. If you see just one doctor, he might use one or two in succession before referring you to a back specialist. If you visit a doctor at an urgent care center in the meantime, he might give you a different medication that could interact with your first prescription and cause serious problems.

There's no substitute for a primary care physician who knows you. So your best bet is to use urgent care centers as a backup if your primary care provider has trouble squeezing you in. Just be sure to notify your primary care office about any new medications or instructions you're given.

Navigating the Doctor's Office

While medicine may be about caring for people, medical offices are also about making money. Even an office that looks run-down is expensive to maintain, and costs the same whether one person shows up or a hundred. In order to cover costs and make a living, your doctor wants to see as many patients as possible. And yes, he'd rather waste your time than his.

That's why you sit in the waiting room until an exam room opens up, and that's why you sit in an exam room while the doctor is with another patient. Because of basic laws of economics, you will never get around the waiting element in the doctor's office unless you find a doctor who has no patients. In that case, if he's any good, expect your luck to run out as soon as word gets out and the practice fills up.

You can, however, mitigate the time spent waiting by asking for an appointment first thing in the morning, or right before the doctor's office closes. If there's no one ahead of you in the morning, the cumulative effect of dozens of late visits has yet to materialize. At the end of the day, your doctor is playing catch-up so he can get home on time. This may mean a shorter visit, but it also means shorter waits.

Neither of these tactics works perfectly—if your doctor's office is attached to a hospital, he may have responsibilities there, or meetings may throw off his schedule. To avoid unplanned waits, call ahead and check how close your doctor's office is to running on schedule. Best to find out that there's an hour wait time before you end up looking at that 1998 *Redbook* all afternoon.

Asking Questions

If you have any specific requests or complaints, you should voice them at the beginning of the exam, so your doctor can take them into account and examine you or order tests accordingly. Even questions about a certain drug you saw advertised on TV–*even if you don't need that drug*–are helpful to your doctor because the questions tip him off that you're concerned about yeast infections, high cholesterol, migraines, insomnia, or whatever else you bring up.

The easiest way to break the awkwardness of asking questions is to write down any questions you have the night before, or while you're in the waiting room. Then you can pull out your card and say "I had a few questions I wanted to ask you." As the Boy Scouts say, "be prepared." You wouldn't go into a meeting unprepared, and your health is just as important as proofreading your stack of PowerPoint slides.

Your Medical Records

Like the mythical "permanent record" from school days, medical records always inspire worries. Medical information is sensitive; no one wants their bad habits to become part of the public record. Speaking about these things is scary enough without imagining someone digging through the information without your consent.

If there's something you're really concerned about having in writing, you can always ask, before you mention it, if your doctor would agree not to write it down. Although we learn in medical school to take notes on everything, many doctors will comply with your wishes as long as this particular bit of information isn't critical to your care.

If your doctor won't agree to go off the record, then you should understand what happens to any notes your doctor takes during your visit. These papers stay in your doctors' folders, and (aside from your insurer, which I'll address below) they should only be shared with other medical personnel for the purposes of providing your care. That means that not only does anyone asking for your folder need to be a medical professional, that person also needs to have a reason for asking.

While these files are basically secure, secretaries and others in your doctor's office will have access. If that bothers you, or if your sister-in-law is the office manager, keep it in mind.

Other than medical professionals, your records can only be obtained by you, your insurer, and anyone to whom you give written permission. If you are paying cash for your visit, then the records are truly yours. Health insurance companies audit your information for only two reasons: to document a preexisting condition, and to audit your doctor's office's billing procedures.

Insurance companies call me on occasion to ask about records because a new client will claim a new diagnosis, and they want to confirm whether it's new or preexisting. Often, all they can do is ask for your doctors' names so they can ask for your records.

If you're asking an insurer to pay for your care, then the insurer does have a stake in your providing truthful information. But if you're terribly concerned about confidentiality, and you're paying cash, you don't have to give any identifying information at the doctor's office. They don't ask you to show ID, and they won't check your background before seeing you. As long as you have a plan in place to follow up on results, either in person or on the telephone, you certainly have the right to withhold personal information.

Public Health Authorities

Now, for some positive test results such as syphilis or tuberculosis, the local health authorities will want to contact you after the results are in. By law, the labs report these results directly to the health authorities, so you have no say in their finding out. The bureau of public health will want to know when it's most likely you were exposed, and get a list of all the people you could have spread the disease to. The public health authorities will also want to ensure that you are getting treated so you don't pass the disease to someone else in the future.

Like most things in medicine, this is all voluntary reporting. I've seen people get the call from the bureau of public health in New York, and blow it off completely. When you get right down to it, these officials are only interested in serving the public good by limiting the spread of disease. They are counting on you to feel the same way, and while they can't compel you to comply, basic humanity and decency should prevail over self-interest when it comes to serious medical problems.

While this process may seem like a deterrent to going in to get tested, it really shouldn't be. The information doesn't go back to your employer or insurer; all the public health department does is track down the people who were exposed so you don't have to. They also keep sexual partner tracking anonymous, simply saying the person was exposed, not who exposed him or her. Once the authorities do their job and make sure that you and everyone else have been treated, they are no longer involved and the record is buried somewhere away from prying eyes.

Life Insurance

Health insurance companies and public health authorities aren't the only ones in the business who have an interest in your medical records. Some life insurance companies require you to get an initial physical as part of the policy (others don't, so read the fine print if you care). If your policy requires a visit, in most cases they'll hook you up with a physician the plan works with who will draw blood to check for various conditions. You'll likely be checked for HIV and undergo the same comprehensive screening that your own physician would recommend on an annual basis.

I've gotten a few phone calls from patients who have had surprisingly high cholesterol levels on these tests, or who are concerned that they might "fail" their insurance physicals and end up with higher premiums. Here are a few tips that will help you avoid a surprise:

- **Get an "unofficial" physical from your own doctor first.** About a third of people in this country have high blood pressure, and most don't even know it. Elevated blood pressure, high cholesterol, or a family history of heart disease could raise your premiums. Treating these conditions won't lower your premiums, but at least you'll know what you're up against.

- **Do all your blood work fasting.** Too many people forget to avoid all food for eight hours before the test. Miss this step, and that cheeseburger you had for lunch might make your cholesterol levels look like you're a step away from a heart attack. I've had to write more than a few letters to insurers supporting my patients who had the cheeseburger/heart condition test double their premiums.

- **Obtain your medical records and look them over before submitting them.** Your insurance company is going to base your policy on what it hears from your physician. If your doctor has made an error or is not up to date on your lifestyle (for instance, you've stopped drinking recently) you need to identify this and address it with your physician before that information lands in the insurance company's lap. Flip through your medical records and ask yourself "What would I be worried about if I were going to insure me?" If you would be concerned, your insurance company will be, too.

If you take these few simple steps, your insurance company will have an accurate view of your risk and will set your premiums accordingly. While some life insurance problems can be fixed after the fact, it's better to be prepared than have a miscommunication cost you some serious cash.

The Healthy Guide to *Healthy* Living

All the insurance industry bureaucracy and all my healthy tips for unhealthy living come down to one thing: When you were little, your parents may have forced you to go to the doctor and take care of your health needs, but once you've grown up, this is up to you.

You don't want to spend any more time in the medical system than you need to. While there are plenty of ways to indulge your bad habits in a more healthful manner, the best way to avoid medical trouble, and to keep your health expenses and life insurance premiums low, is to take a few simple precautions. If you take nothing else from this book, copy this page. These healthy tips for healthy living will make you feel better and live longer than anything else:

1. Exercise.

2. Quit smoking soon—preferably *NOW*.

3. Eat like your body matters.

4. Drink a little alcohol, but not too much.

5. Gentlemen: Wear a condom when you have sex;
   Ladies: Make sure he does, and use birth control, too.

6. Limit your partners, and keep the ones you have happy.

7. Get enough sleep.

8. Surround yourself with supportive, positive people.

9. Deal with life head-on, not through a drug-induced haze.

10. Never be afraid to change your life for the better.

Take care of your body and it will take care of you. All the medical miracles in the world and all the tips for healthy unhealthy living I can offer you can't change that truth.

Acknowledgments

WHILE internal medicine doctors see a wide range of maladies, we can't be experts on everything. I'm grateful for the assistance of several other medical professionals who shared their expertise with me for this book. I'd especially like to thank Dr. Kurt Hong, a weight-loss and nutrition expert at UCLA; Dr. Astrid Pujari of the Pujari Center in Seattle, Washington, for her assistance with herbal supplements; and Dr. John Espinola, for his medical editing skills.

I am grateful to my friend Jonathan Steinberg for inspiring me to write *The Healthy Guide to Unhealthy Living* during our trip to Las Vegas in 2002. While what happens in Vegas stays in Vegas, we realized that lots of folks worry about what the Vegas lifestyle can do to their health—and this book is the result.

I'd like to thank my coauthor, Laura Vanderkam, for turning my notes into the book you just read. She'd like to thank her husband, Michael Conway, for dutifully forwarding stories about new drugs and studies, and for understanding the deadline pressures that have writers cranking out copy about binge drinking on their honeymoons.

Laura and I would like to thank our agents, Emily Nurkin and Laura Yorke, both of the Carol Mann Agency in New York, for placing this book with Simon & Schuster. They recognized that *The Healthy Guide to Unhealthy Living* was a great idea for a book, and recognized that we would work well together. They were right.

We'd also like to thank Sydny Miner, senior editor at Simon & Schuster, for her guidance in preparing this manuscript. She reeled us in when we got out of hand, asked the right questions, and made sure we were answering the questions readers would care most about.

Writing a book always requires the support of family and friends, and I'd like to thank all of them for sharing their stories and encouraging this project. Their help made writing *The Healthy Guide to Unhealthy Living* a lot more fun.

Index